Novels by Patrick L. Deu Pree

Kshatriya, the Legend of Nathaniel J. Smith
Kshatriya II, Captain Steel
Reign of the Golden Goddess
The Angel and the Hitman
Apocalypse Dawn
Jiang Li, River Beautiful
Steel Gray
Black Jade
Black Jade II, Redemption
Black Jade III, Full Pardon
Deputy Ronda Miller/The Protector

51 YEARS UNDER THE IRON

BY
PATRICK L. DEU PREE

AN ACTION BOOK

TO MY TEACHER,
CHARLES P. MALLON

TO MY WIFE,
DONNA

Table of Contents

INTRODUCTION

Hi. My name is Patrick L. Deu Pree, otherwise known by my friends as "Pat." That's the name I like to be called by but some people insist on calling me "Patrick"!

Anyway. You probably know me from the action/adventure novels I have written. I've written eleven of them. But I have never shared the fact that I am a personal trainer and a recreational bodybuilder except for a brief author bio on the back of my other books.

I have been training people and training myself for over fifty years now. I had my humble beginnings in 1964 at Charlie Mallon's Physical Culture Studio in San Francisco at the age of 17. I was the skinniest kid that ever walked into Charlie's Gym that fateful day. This book describes my personal journey and also outlines training programs that I have discovered that can be of help to average people trying to stay in shape. There are also programs for building as much muscle mass one can acquire in a natural way. I disdain steroids and always have. I have never used them. Whatever gains I made I made with hard work and proper eating. And, proper rest, a factor not discussed as deeply as I am going to discuss it. So, I welcome you on this journey and I hope you will learn something that will be of value in your life.

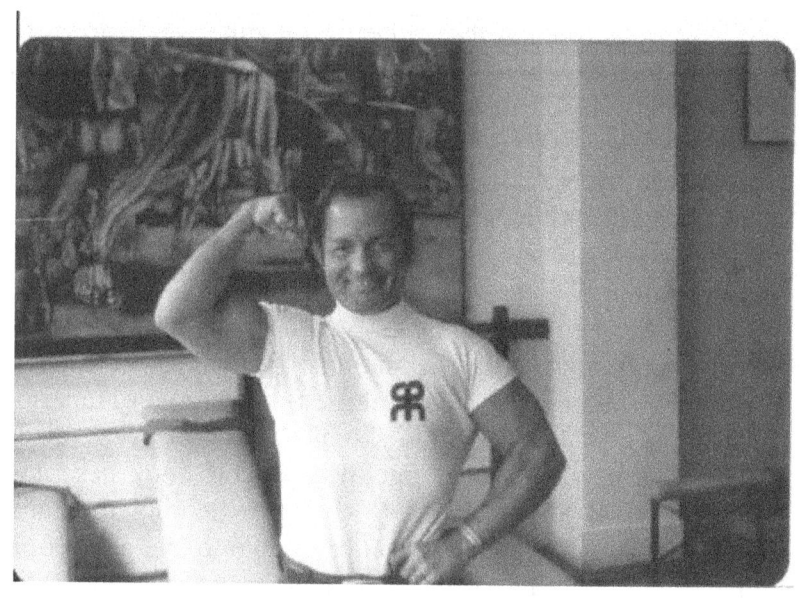

My teacher, Charles P. Mallon.

CHAPTER ONE
"HUMBLE BEGINNINGS"

I remember it like it was just yesterday. The day I first walked into Charlie Mallon's Physical Culture Studio at 256 Sutter Street, San Francisco, California. 2nd floor.

This very built but very short man came walking swiftly across the training room floor and shook my hand. This was my introduction to Charlie Mallon. He was to become a great, lifelong friend.

But I was just a dumb kid at the time with visions of becoming the next bodybuilding champion. I worshiped all the top bodybuilders like Larry Scott, God rest his soul, and Dave Draper. There were other big names, Chuck Sipes, Freddy Ortiz to name a few.

My first inspiration came when I was 12 years old. That summer I saw the movie *HERCULES* starring Steve Reeves. It totally blew my mind. At 12 I was already 6'1 ½" and weighed only 120 pounds. I was the weakest kid in school. I lived many of my days in fear of other, bigger kids who would torment and push me around. Seeing the movie *HERCULES* gave me a vision of how I wanted to be. I searched and searched for the answer.

I had other physical ailments and the doctors told my mother that I should never ever do any strenuous physical activities. It would "strain my heart."

Thus, I felt there was no hope. But I never lost the burning desire to gain solid muscle and stand with the other kids, being accepted by them finally. I was an outcast. I wrote stories and comic books, heroic adventure stories and the main hero always was built like a bodybuilder. Thus was my first foray into writing fiction. Little did I know where it would eventually lead.

So there I stood, in Charlie Mallon's gym. The first thing he did was to take my measurements. I had a 32" chest, 10" arms, 27" inch waist and 15" thighs.

He started me out on the beginner's routine:

Bench Press   3x7
Squats   3x15
Supersetted with straight armed pullovers on the flat bench. 15 reps.
Bent Over Rows 3x7
Upright Row   3x7
Curls   3x7

This was the basic routine for gaining muscle mass I followed. He also had me taking health drinks, mixtures of eggs. There was one drink called "the green drink" which consisted of orange juice, avocado and honey. This I drank prior to my workout.

Charlie taught me to breathe deeply in all my exercises. Especially the squats. He had me superset the squats with straight arm pullovers. In otherwords, I would do the pullovers immediately after finishing a set of squats without rest in between. This was to expand my rib cage for I had a very caved in look to my chest. I worked out Monday, Wednesday and Friday. I would take the bus over to San Francisco from Mill Valley, where I lived. I would catch the bus right out in front of Tamalpias High School where I went to school.

That year I put on thirty pounds of muscle. My chest went from 32" to 40", my arms, from 10" to 12" and my thighs went from 15" to 19". My waist went to 29".

Although still considered skinny, I had muscles. And I was

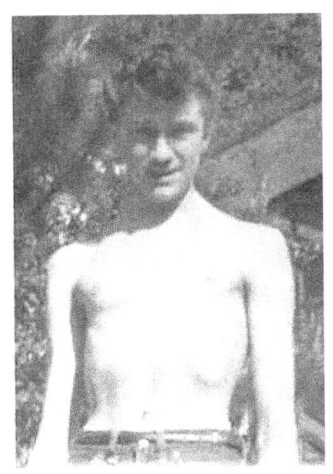

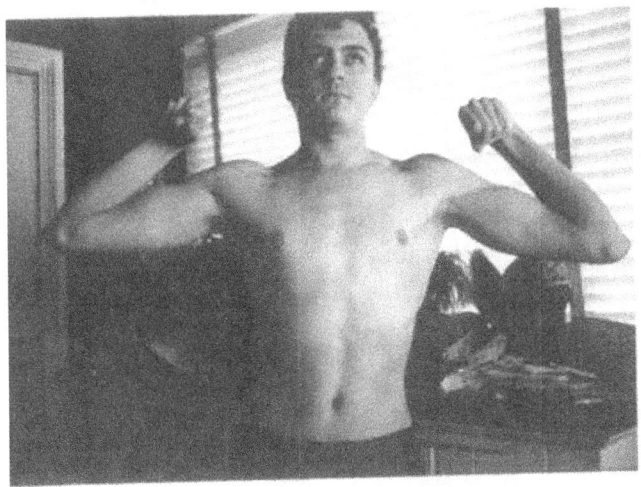

At 17 and a year later at 18 and 30 pounds heaiver.

standing up for myself more against certain bullies in high school. I would flex my muscles in the mirror and was amazed. I had flaring lats, my biceps were rounded.

I hit my workout routines with a vengeance and read everything I could find in the muscle magazines. The main muscle magazines in those days were *MUSCLE BUILDER, MR. AMERICA, STRENTH AND HEALTH* and a new publication, *MUSCULAR DEVELOPMENT*. And of course, *IRON MAN MAGAZINE* published by Peary Rader.

MR. AMERICA and *MUSCLE BUILDER* were both Weider publications and were filled with the pictures of the top bodybuilding champions of the day. Larry Scott and Dave Draper. They were the winners of the IFBB titles, MR. AMERICA and MR. UNIVERSE.

STRENGTH AND HEALTH and *MUSCULAR DEVELOPMENT* were both publications by Bob Hoffman who was violently opposed to Joe Weider. I didn't really care about that, what I wanted was to be strong. That's all, just to be big and strong.

So I filled my head with everything I could find on gaining strength and muscle. I am a hard gainer, I was soon to find out, and every pound of muscle was hard earned. Over the years I eventually put on seventy pounds, taking myself up to 190 lbs with a 46" chest. Wow! From a 32" chest to a 46" chest! It really blew my mind.

But this journey took many years. In the following chapters I will show you shortcuts you can take that I have learned to gain as much muscle size as possible.

CHAPTER TWO
"THE HARD GAINER"

As I have said, I am a hard gainer. I am the classic ectomorph. Small, thin, very long bones. This is why the doctors said I should never train with weights and why they said it was impossible for me to gain muscle mass. I instinctively knew different. And I had the burning desire to succeed. So I hit my training routines with a vengeance and after many years I succeeded. Actually, I hit 170 lbs at 25 but couldn't hold it. I had taken up martial arts and with all the aerobic activity I found it was very difficult to gain any size. It was a conflict. I will deal with that later. If you really want the most in muscle size and you are naturally skinny like I was then you have to specialize.

Weight training is the basis for all athletic activity though. A strong body is a capable body. There is no such thing as "muscle bound". That is an absolute myth. When I combined martial arts with weight training I only benefited.

But like I said, I am a hard gainer. I would eat the amount of food a 200 lb man would eat and only weigh 145 lbs. It seemed almost impossible. But I finally succeeded as the photos will show you.

When you are a hard gainer you have to concentrate on a basic routine. Bench presses, squats, rowing, military presses, deadlifts. These are the exercises that place the most demand on the body and cause it, with proper nutrition and rest, to grow. Especially rest. Recuperation is the name of this game. Get enough sleep at night, at least seven or eight hours. And enough food. Drink a lot of whole milk if you can. If you are

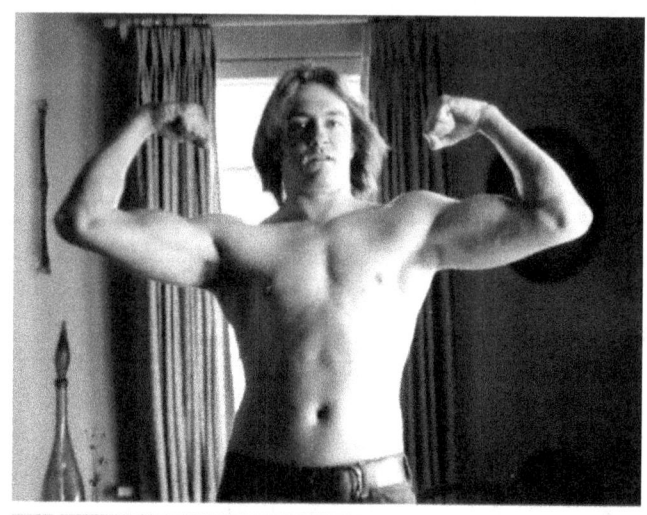

At 25 years of age.

lactose intolerant which I now am, then you can now use lactose free milk. There are many options out there today that there never used to be.

Milk and egg protein supplements are also an aid to gaining muscle mass. If you drink a gallon of milk with a level cup of milk and egg protein or whey protein mixed into it you will definitely gain muscle mass very quickly. I will give you formulas that will help you.

If you don't get enough sleep you can lose as much as five pounds.

The question arises, what about someone with no time to train, the busy person who has to work long hours then help with the family?

I have found ways around this so the busiest person can train hard and make good progress in gaining size and muscle mass and maintaining it once it has been gained. The following chapters will deal with this. We all have to work for a living but that is no excuse not to train. All it takes is desire.

CHAPTER THREE
"DESIRE"

It is one thing to want to improve. It is another to actually do it. You really have to want it with everything in your being to succeed. I had that desire. I hated the way I was and I trained my heart out to succeed. I had the burning desire. That's what you have to have or you will fall right on your face. There is no other way around this. If you look in the mirror and hate what you see, then you have to have a strong enough will to succeed. Half measures won't do it. I have seen many people start to train, work out maybe a week and then never come back. Those people just didn't want it bad enough.

What about young people working and also going to school? I made a big mistake when I was young. I sacrificed a college education because I was too dedicated to my training. I later realized that I could have done both. Body building champion Larry Scott worked full time, trained hard, and went to night school. And he was one of the greatest bodybuilding champions who ever lived. He also considered himself a hard gainer. But he did it and had a great career and acquired great wealth.

I will show you specialized routines that you can do that fit into a busy schedule. That's why I wrote this book. This is not a book for advanced bodybuilders who are interested in bodybuilding competition. This is for men and women of average or below average genetics. Anyone can improve. As far as being a bodybuilding champion, perhaps one person in 100,000 has the genetic ability to put on that kind of muscle mass. I wasted a lot time trying to become what I never could become. Train hard and eat right and let your body grow to its potential.

What is your particular potential? Only you will be able to find that out. A general guide line is that if you are an extreme ectomorph like I was, then perhaps you will never have the ability to become a champion. But you may have the hidden genetic ability. A bodybuilder named Joe Dodd, in the seventies, build a massive physique and won many titles. When he began training he only had 11" arms, was skinny as a rail yet, he succeeded. His arms eventually measured 19 inches. You never know. Though I never had that ability I still did put on seventy pounds of muscle. Who would have ever known that a six foot one and a half one hundred and twenty pound kid would eventually weigh one hundred and ninety pounds of solid muscle? Yet I was able to do so.

So, let's get started.

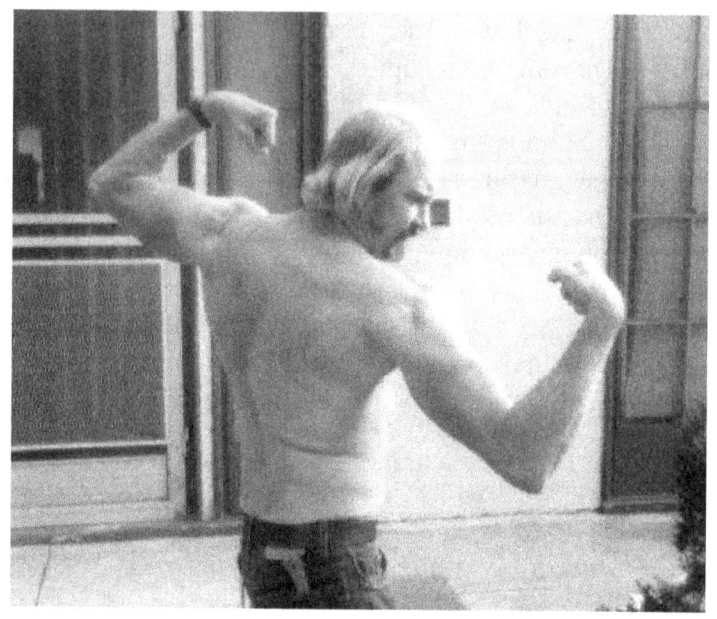

At 37 in 1984 and 190 pounds

CHAPTER FOUR
"GETTING STARTED"

Getting started.

The first thing you will need is proper equipment. Or a good gym. There are certain key pieces of equipment that are absolutely mandatory. These are a bench with racks, a bench without racks, a squat rack, and an adjustable barbell and dumbbell set. These are absolutely mandatory. There are no exceptions. Another choice is a heavy duty bench with no racks and a power cage. With a power cage you can do many different exercises. Squats, bench presses, military presses off the racks, etc.

If you have no room for this equipment then join a local gym. There are many good choices to choose from these days. Gold's Gyms are always a good choice, they have really heavy duty basic equipment as well as machines. I am not opposed to machines but I prefer free weights. In fact I feel that with the basic movements like squats, bench presses and deadlifts that free weights must always be used whenever possible. There are at times exceptions but we will deal with that later.

The next thing you will need is a weight lifting belt. Make sure it is no wider than four inches in back. Any more than that will be placing too much support on the muscles of the torso. You want protection from injury but you want to make sure the muscles are worked as well. Wear loose clothing that will not hinder your movement. A sweat shirt and sweat pants are a good example. Always make sure the muscles are covered especially on cold days. Arnold Schwarzenegger once told me back in 1972 at the original Gold's Gym in Venice that it was vitally important to keep the muscles warm so you would not incur an injury. I have always obeyed this rule.

A word on home equipment. The Bowflex machine is a great machine for home workouts. You can do all the basic movements with it. But if you have a spare room and can get a bench, weights and squat rack in it, that's even better. Buy a couple of floor mats if you have to to protect the carpeting if you are in an apartment.

If you have a house with a garage, that's perfect. Or a back yard patio setup. I have my weights and equipment in my garage. I have a lot of stuff stored in there but I have made a space for my workouts. You don't need a lot of space, about eight feet by eight feet works really well. I've actually seen weight equipment set up in apartment living rooms. Whatever works.

Now you are ready for the workout routine.

CHAPTER FIVE
"THE WORKOUT"

The workout is a very simple, basic routine. It almost may seem too simple. It isn't, believe me. The workout will be the hardest thing you've ever done physically. It's supposed to be that way.

We will use the basics listed below:

Bench Press

Squats

Still Legged or Romanian Deadlift

Barbell or Dumbbell rows

Military Presses

Curls

Lying Triceps Extensions

Ab, neck and forearm work

Those are the nuts and bolts of the program. There are many other exercises but these are "secondary" exercises and we are not going to dwell much on these as they are only used in advanced routines when all the muscle mass has been acquired. Don't concern yourself with these. I will describe an "advanced" routine later. You may never even get to such a routine or even want to. I rarely do such routines. I always stick to the rock bottom basics described above.

This routine will be done twice a week with several days in between for rest and recuperation. The workout can be divided up as follows: Monday and Thursday, Tuesday and Friday, Wednesday and Saturday. Get the idea? You need the days in between for rest and recuperation. When you lift weights you break down, destroy, muscle tissue. The body then, with proper rest and eating, builds back up, repairs the damage and adds more muscle for protection. That's how muscle is built.

You will do a warm up set before each exercise with a light weight then do two sets of each exercise for six to twelve repetitions. No more than that. It's not volume that builds muscle, it's intensity. Two hard sets are perfect for this, especially in the beginning. I never do more than two sets. It's how hard you work each set.

Proper breathing.

It's important to breathe properly when working out. Think of oxygen as energy. You fill your lungs with energy before executing intense effort. For example, on the bench press, take the bar off the racks and hold it overhead. Take in a deep breath then lower the weight to your chest. Then, as you lift the weight, breathe out powerfully! That's how it works. The oxygen in your blood gives you energy! Always remember to breathe properly.

This is especially important when doing squats. When doing squats, take a deep breath before lowering yourself into the deep squat position then let the breath explode out as you drive upwards. Do this for the first couple of reps. Then, you should be really tired. For the next couple of reps, take two breaths before going into the squat, then three or four breaths. The squat is the number one exercise in this program. It is the key to all progress. It is called "the king of the exercises" and rightly so. You'll see that after you do a hard set of squats, you should feel like you have run into a brick wall. If you don't, you haven't been doing the exercise hard enough.

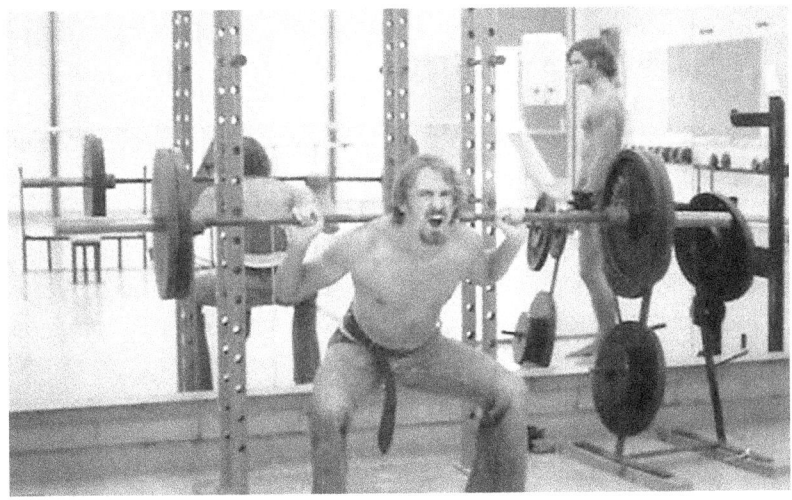

Squats are the key to the program!

CHAPTER SIX
"MORE ABOUT SQUATS"

As I said in the last chapter, squats are the key to this entire program. There are really no substitutes. Squats are number one. Heavy squats cause the body to grow. It ups fat burning, causes a heavy demand on the body to build more muscle, not just in the legs, but for the entire body.

When I was 27 years old I was working out in the weight room at Marin College. I had just finished a heavy set of squats and had set the bar back on the racks of the power cage. One of the football coaches came walking in, seeing me he said, "Of course, young man, you must realize you won't be doing squats after you're thirty."

Well, coach, I'm almost seventy now, and guess what?

That's right. I am still doing squats as part of my regular training program.

Doing squats took me eventually from 120 pounds to 190 pounds. It took many years but it worked. From what I have learned I have streamlined the program so one can achieve that goal and more in a much shorter time.

Squats cause the body to produce more natural testosterone and growth hormone. Needed elements in producing muscle mass. The added testosterone gives one a greater sense of well being, for both men and women. It strengthens bones, a very important thing as we get older. My doctor, looking over my blood work when I was in my early sixties said, "You have the blood work of a teenager."

So never make up excuses for not doing squats in your

weight training program.

Are there any substitutes? What if you have a bad back? There are ways to work around that, you can do 45 degree leg presses and get almost the same result. But be careful on the leg presses, they can also strain the lower back. Always pay perfect attention to proper form.

I am not going to lie to you. This is a hard program. It takes will power. But you are reaching for excellence, for improvement. Otherwise you would never have purchased this book. Am I correct?

Thought so.

Now I am going to talk for a bit about will power.

CHAPTER SEVEN
"WILL POWER"

These days no one talks much about will power. It's not considered politically correct. It's said that one has "emotional issues". Not a lack of will power.

I am here to tell you that that's a bunch of nonsense. You need will power to survive in the world, not just to train. You exercise will power every time you get up to go to work in the morning, facing a hard job. It takes will power.

Will power is doing that which is hard, no matter what. You don't work out "just when it feels right". You work out when you are scheduled to do so, no matter what. Illness is an exception to that rule. If you are sick, then what you need is rest. Or if you are recovering from an injury.

Back when I was young, in the late sixties, I got involved in a lot of things I should never have become involved in. Those things sapped my will power and I was missing workouts. I lost much of my hard earned gains. A motorcycle accident brought me back to my senses. As I lay in the hospital bed with a broken foot I swore I'd change things. Recovery was hard. I had to learn to walk all over again. But I healed and then returned to Charlie Mallon's Gym and began training again with a vengeance. There were days I just didn't want to go in to work out. But I forced myself and always felt better. I rebuilt my lost muscle mass and went on to add much more.

It was because I used will power. I trained no matter what. And it's the same thing with writing. I would never have written and published eleven novels had I not practiced will power. Even in the writing of this book, there are days I have to really force myself to open my laptop.

Will power.

It's built by doing things that are hard.

Being Selfish

Be selfish! You heard me right! Be selfish. You have a right to take care of yourself. I have met people who are always "doing for others". Never taking time for themselves. In being selfish I don't mean to be completely self obsessed. We are all interconnected and have the responsibility to look after each other, to a point.

But I have seen cases where someone is always looking out for everyone else and taking no time to take care of themselves. Forget working out. They "never have time"; there is always something they have to do. Others take advantage of them and suck up all their energy.

Set boundaries! If you don't take time for yourself you will certainly come to deeply regret it. You have to take care of yourself or one day you will be old and broken down and everyone you thought cared for you will be gone. I have seen this happen too many times.

Always take time out for working out, for meditation and just for "alone time" for yourself. This is mental health. This is self care. You deserve, remember that! There are workouts in this book that can be done in a short amount of time. Make time to take care of yourself. It may be difficult at first. Others will resent you not being there for them 24/7. These people are energy vampires and will suck the life out of you. They don't give a rat's ass about you. Talk about being selfish?

When you insist on time for yourself they will be resentful and some will leave.

Good!

You don't need these people in your life! As you embark of a course of improving yourself others will come into your life who will respect you. Because you are taking care of yourself you will find others who will give you positive reinforcement.

I know of someone who was so involved in caring for others that when she thought about taking even ten minutes to meditate they heaped all kinds of guilt on her. Don't be like this person! A workout life style is a positive action and as you progress you will draw more positive relationships into your life.

Always take time for yourself. No one cares about you like you!

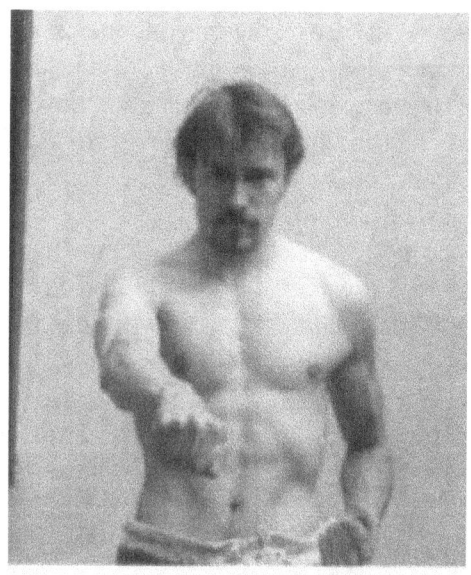

A strong will helped me in the
Practice of karate.

CHAPTER EIGHT
"PERFORMING THE EXERCISES"

Now we get to the real deal here. The actual exercises. I am going to describe each of the necessary exercises needed in this program. These are the core basic exercises you will need.

First the warmup.

Ab Crunch

The first exercise is the ab crunch. While lying on the floor on a carpet or exercise mat with knees bent, hands folded across your chest or behind your head, curl your upper torso forward towards your knees. This is not a sit up. I do not recommend sit ups as they strain the hips and low back. Rather, the safer way to work the upper abs is with the ab crunch. In my own workout area I use an exercise mat and a device called the ab roller. But you can work the abs without the ab roller. Do fifty repetition of this exercise.

Leg Raise off Bench

The next exercise is the leg raise off the bench. Sit on the edge of a bench and bring your knees up towards your chest. Always bend your legs. Never do ab crunches or leg raises with straight legs as this is hazardous to your lower back. It's safer done with bent knees. The idea is to stress the upper and lower abs, not to cause an injury. Do fifty repetitions.

Good Mornings

This exercise will warm up the lower back and rear thighs. Place a light weight, no heavier than 25 to 45 pounds, across the back of your shoulders, not the back of your neck. Now, bend forward until your torso is horizontal to the floor and then raise back up to the standing position. Do this 20 times.

Now you are warmed up and ready to do the rest of the workout.

Bench Press

The king of the upper body exercises. Lying flat on the bench, grip the bar wider than shoulder width apart and take the bar off the stands, holding it over your head. While holding the weight over your head take a deep breath. Now lower the weight until it touches your mid chest. While breathing out strongly, raise the weight back up to arm's length. Do 12 repetitions to begin with.

Barbell Squats

The overall king of all the exercises! This is the number one growth producing exercise for the entire body as well as a fantastic leg developer.

Face the rack, get under the bar, letting it ride across the back of your shoulders. Step out from the rack with your feet a little wider than shoulder width apart, toes facing outward. Now, take a deep breath. With knees going in the direction of your toes, squat down until you thighs are parallel or slightly below parallel to the floor. Now, drive back up to the standing position while breathing out strongly. Repeat for twelve repetitions.

The Stiff Legged Deadlift

Sometimes called the Romanian Deadlift, this exercise is also an overall growth producer as well as a fantastic exercise for your lower back and rear thighs, also for your trapezius muscles, the large muscle group extending down from your neck to your shoulders. It also works your grip. In fact, if you have trouble holding the bar you may want to use a reverse grip, one hand gripping the bar with palm facing inward and the other hand with the palm facing outward. Bending the knees, raise the bar off the floor and hold it waist high. Take a deep breath. Now, with only a very slight bend of the knees, bend forward, riding the bar close to the body, down the thighs to mid shin. That's far enough. Now, breathing out strongly, raise back up to the standing position, shrugging the shoulders at the top of the movement. Repeat for 12 repetitions then return the barbell to the floor. If using a power cage, you can set the bar on low racks about midway between the thighs rather than taking the bar off the floor for the beginning of the exercise.

Bent Over Rows or Single Dumbbell Rows

You can use one or the other of these exercises but not both. They strongly work the back, the latissimus dorsi muscles, one of the largest muscle groups of the upper body. It builds "wide lats."

Bent Over Rows With Barbell

Bend over at the waist, back straight and slightly arched. Grip the barbell on the floor at a slightly wider than shoulder grip. Bend the knees slightly and hold the weight so it is several inches from the floor. Now, take a deep breath and lift the weight until the bar touches the lower chest while breathing out strongly. Then lower the weight and repeat. Do 12 repetitions then return the weight to the floor.

The Dumbbell Row

This works the same muscle area but the lower back does not come into play here. I use this exercise as the result of back injuries rather than the regular barbell row. I suggest that everyone over thirty switch to this way of working the lats.

Place a dumbbell next to a bench. Bend forward, placing one hand on the bench and grip the dumbbell with the other hand. Lift the weight so it is several inches from the floor. Now, take a deep breath. While breathing out strongly, lift the dumbbell so it touches your lower chest then lower the weight back down several inches from the floor. Repeat for 12 repetitions then set the dumbbell back on the floor. Repeat with the other hand on the bench. This is one set.

The Standing Military Press

If you are working in a power cage or a squat rack, place the holds at chest level and set the bar on the racks. Otherwise, hoist the barbell from the floor and hold at chest height. Take a deep breath. Now, while breathing out strongly, press the bar overhead to arms length. Then lower the weight back to chest level while breathing in. Repeat for 12 repetitions.

The Barbell Regular Curl

This is the main biceps builder. Stand with bar held at arm's length. Take a deep breath. While breathing out strongly, curl the weight all the way up until it touches your chest. Then return the bar to arms length and repeat for 12 repetitions.

Lying Triceps Extension

This is the main exercise for building the triceps, the large muscle group opposite the biceps. In fact, to build really large arms, the main bulk of the arms are the triceps.

Lie down on the bench holding the bar with a close grip over your head. Breathe in deeply and lower the weight by bending the elbows down behind your head. Now, breathing out strongly, lift the weight by straightening the arms until the weight is again over your head. Repeat for 12 repetitions.

There you have it!

That's the basic barbell routine that builds a fantastic body for both men and women! Do this routine twice a week and you will get great results! If you are on a busy schedule you can do this routine once a week and still get great results. In fact, I have used a similar routine for years once a week and maintained myself in great shape.

I will discuss this in the next chapter.

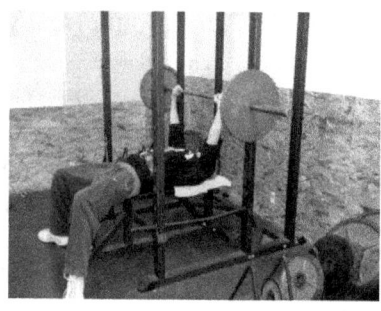

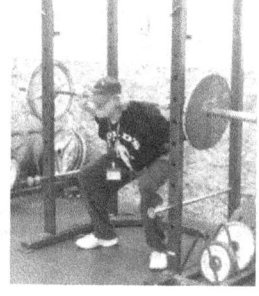

BENCH PRESS   *SQUATS*

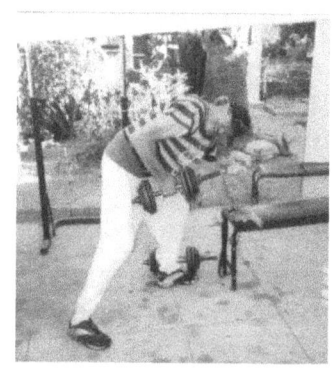

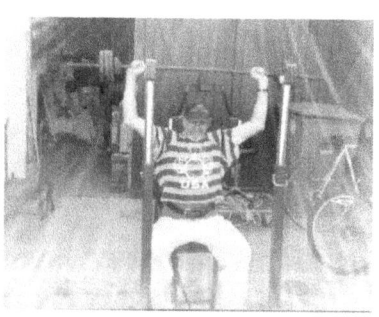

DUMBBELL ROW   *SEATED MILITARY PRESS*

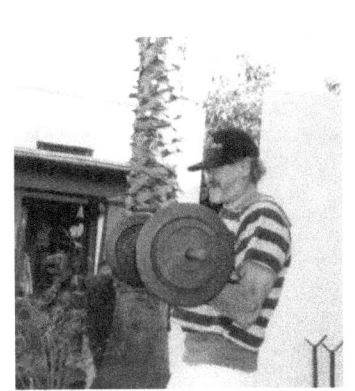 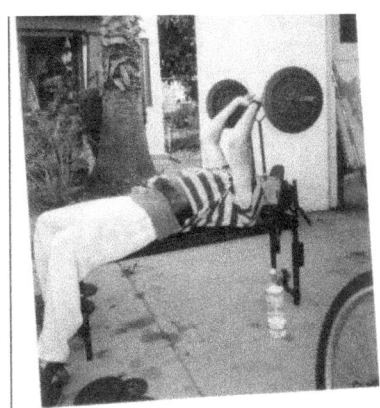

CURLS   *LYING TRICEPS EXTENSIONS*

CHAPTER NINE
"THE ONCE A WEEK WORKOUT"

Work out once a week? Are you crazy?

Back in 1975 I had a back room gym at my house where I would train and would also train a few select friends. I always, at that time, worked out three times a week, Monday, Wednesday and Friday, right after getting off work. On Tuesday and Thursday I would train on the martial arts at my sensei, Gus Johnson's dojo. I lived in Mill Valley, California and the dojo was just north in San Rafael.

A friend of mine, Dave Kong, was a student at that time at San Francisco State College where he was working on his Master's in sociology. He felt he was not getting enough out of his free hand workout, mainly push ups and situps which he would do every morning before taking the bus from Mill Valley to San Francisco to school. I had been trying to convince him to come workout at my gym but he would say that he just didn't have enough time to work out with weights.

One day he came over while I was taking a workout and he said he wanted to train at my gym but he would only have the time to work out on Fridays. That was only once a week, I said. I told him I didn't really believe that he could get any real results from training only once a week and that it was mandatory that he work out three times a week, minimum.

Dave insisted that he could only work out once a week on Fridays so I said, "Okay, go ahead and give it a shot but I really don't think it will work."

So every Friday he would come by and I would coach him.

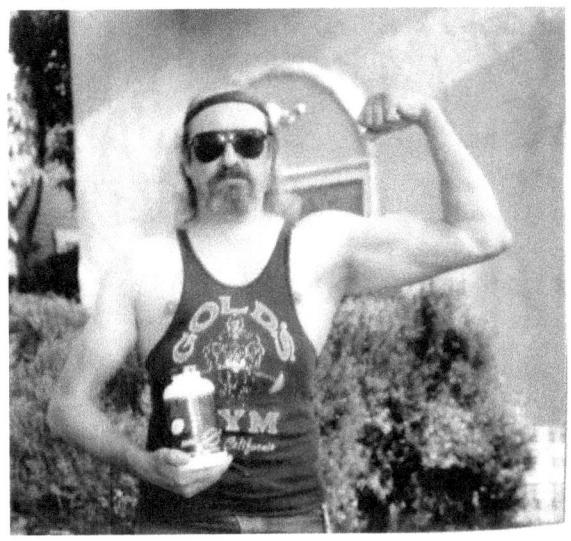

I put more mass on working out once a week then I ever had before!

Was I in for a surprise! In six months he had greatly improved his build, had added much muscle mass and strength! It actually worked! Dave Kong worked out once a week and made great gains in strength and muscle!

I still worked out three times a week until 1978 when I moved down to Los Angeles.

When I got to Los Angeles I did construction labor and was quite exhausted. I was working out at Gold's Gym in Santa Monica at that time. This is before Gold's became a big franchise and there was only one Gold's Gym and that was on Second Street in Santa Monica. When I had first arrived in Los Angeles that summer I had some cash so I trained three times a week there and then I would hit the beach at Venice. But within three weeks I had to find work so I did construction labor which was exhausting. So I would hit Gold's on Saturday mornings and I found it worked.

In later years as I had a busier and busier schedule I worked out once a week and found I made greater gains than I ever had before.

This game is based on recuperation. When you work out you destroy muscle tissue. Then, during the rest phase, your body repairs the damage by building back up and then over compensating by adding even more muscle to take on the demand that was placed upon the body.

By resting for a week in between hard workouts you maximize your recuperation. So a once a week workout works very well. It would be nice if we could just go to the gym every day and hit the beach without a care in the world but life doesn't work that way, unless you win the lotto. We do actually have to work and if we're smart, go to school as well. But you don't have to sacrifice your workouts to do this. So a basic, hard workout routine as I have outlined in the former chapter will take care of the problem of staying in shape.

Give it try if you find you're too busy to hit the gym every day or even three times a week.

CHAPTER TEN
"WEIGHT TRAINING AND THE MARTIAL ARTS"

Weight training and martial arts are a fantastic combination. They highly complement each other. As well as working out with weights, I also was intensely involved in karate for a number of years. But I never stopped training with weights. There were a lot of myths abounding concerning weights. The main myth was the old "muscle bound" myth. The fear that training with weights would make one unable to move. That is an absolute myth, a total untruth. There is no such thing as "muscle bound". I have seen some of the most massively built bodybuilders in the entire world, world champion bodybuilders, and I have never ever seen anyone who was muscle bound! There is no such thing!

I have seen some of the most massively muscled men do the total splits, able to touch the floor with the palms of their hands without bending their knees.

A good example is Jean Claude Van Damme. A fantastic martial artist, moves with the speed of lightening, can do the full splits, total flexibility and he is also a bodybuilder with massive, defined muscles.

There is no such thing as "muscle bound". Forget that idea.

When I was involved in martial arts this is the one myth that I had to fight constantly. I always kept my weight training secret because of all the things other martial artists would say if they knew I trained with weights.

My main sensei, Gus Johnson, God rest his soul in Heaven, believed the muscle bound myth and would tell his students that weight training would "slow you down." So I never shared with him that I weight trained.

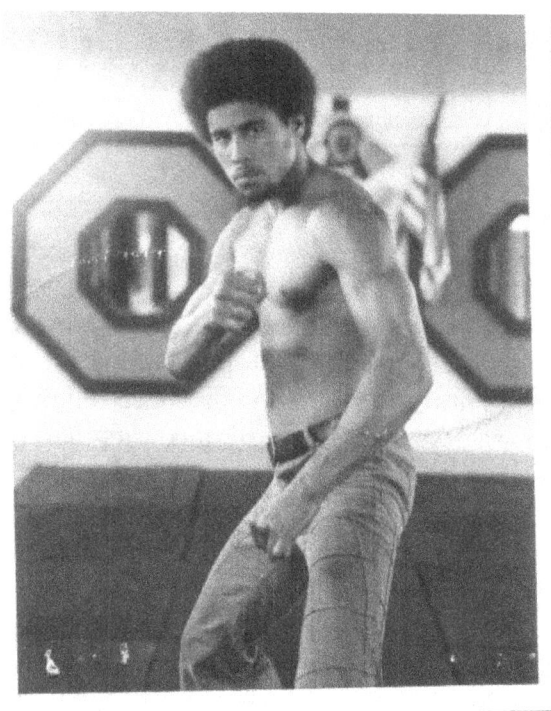

"Mean Gene" Orro, martial artist.

At that time, 1974, I had a fully equipped gym in the back room of my home where I would train myself and some of my friends. On Monday, Wednesday and Friday I would train with weights and on Tuesday and Thursday I would practice karate at Gus Johnson's School of the Dragon.

I met a young man there in November of 1973 when I first started training with Gus Johnson. His name was Gene Orro, Gus's top student. He was of thin but muscular build, similar to me. We got to know each other and I offered to train him on the weights. So he would come by my back room gym and I would train him. And he would teach me martial arts. He grew quickly in strength and added muscle mass. All this we did in secret.

One day in 1975 Gus came by my place, he had heard that I trained people on weights. He had moved the school to a larger location in a basement of an office building in San Rafael, California. He decided he wanted to have a weight training setup in his new school with a qualified instructor. He had heard about me, perhaps Gene had told him, I never actually found out how.

So Pat Deu Pree's Gym was born. It was in a room all to itself, a basic barbell and dumbbell gym. I operated that gym from 1976 to 1978 and trained personally over 200 students at that time. I will discuss this more in a future chapter.

In the 1970s there were no gyms in Marin County. The only place one could train with weights was either at my gym or at the weight room of Marin College, a place where I trained on many occasions. The picture of me on the cover of this book squatting with 225 pounds was taken during the summer of 1974 at the Marin College weight room. I learned many things during the time I operated my own gym at the School of the Dragon and I applied them to my students. I saw that they had great results in both strength and muscle gains. And in martial arts. Some students only wanted to train with weights. One such student was a man named Guy. He was primarily interested in playing softball. He was a car salesman and he was devoted to the game in his spare time. He wanted greater athletic ability and more strength. So I would personally train him three days a week on the basics I have described in the earlier chapter on descriptions of the exercises. He found that right away his ability in his chosen sport was improving. He was so impressed that he brought his younger brother to the gym to work out.

Weight training helps in all other areas of physical

endeavor.

Combining the Two

When I first began martial arts training I was at a loss as to how to combine my passion for weight training with my newfound interest. I was living in the Los Angeles area at that time, in 1972, and was primarily working out at Gold's Gym in Venice. That was in the days when Arnold Schwarzenegger was the top bodybuilding champion of the world. I had talked to him on several occasions and had received some good training advice. But when it came to combining weight training with karate, I was on my own.

I tried to do both on the same day. I was working out with weights three days a week at the time and Young Suh, my first sensei, said that karate had to be practiced every day. No problem on the days I didn't weight train. But on weight training days I had a problem. First I tried to do a karate workout in the morning and then train with weights after work. I was too exhausted. Plus, in karate, the katas, or forms, took up a lot of floor space so I had to go to the dojo as there was no room where I lived to practice them. And the dojo wasn't open at 5:30 in the morning.

I couldn't go out to Gold's Gym, do a full on workout, and then go to the dojo afterwards, Gold's was in Venice and the dojo was in Burbank. There was the Los Angeles freeway system to cope with. At rush hour!

I finally hit on the perfect solution. I was going to give up and I told a massively built bodybuilder at Gold's named Ron Depolito, a good friend of mine. "You can do both," Ron simply said. At that moment I had a realization! I could do both. The answer was right there in front of me.

I'd simply split my training up. Monday, Wednesday and Friday I'd go out to Gold's and train with weights and Tuesday, Thursday and Saturday I'd go to the dojo.

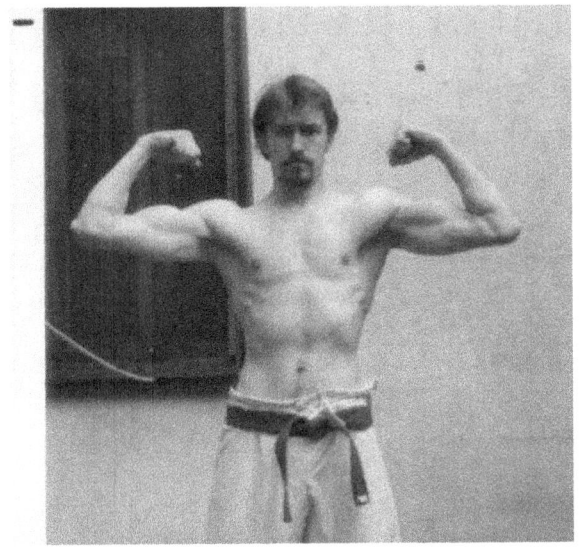

Martial arts added a whole new dimension.

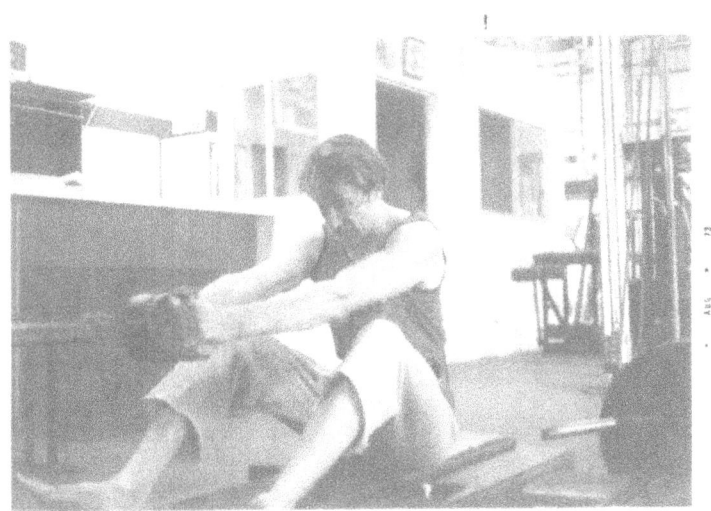

Cable rows at Gold's Gym, 1973. Al Malone photo.

So I tried it and it worked. I could put my full energy into both modes of training that way. I also found that combining both modes of training made me more "cut". I was getting a really streamlined look. Below is the weight training routine I used at that time.

Bench Press	4x8
Squats	4x10
Cable Row	4x8
Standing Military Press	4x8
Barbell Curls	4x8
Lying Triceps Extensions	4x8

I did no ab work at that time because in karate we did a technique called tense and relax. With this technique you tense all the muscles of your body, with emphasis on your lower abdomen. Young Suh had a saying: "When under any kind of stress or challenge, tense lower abdomen!"

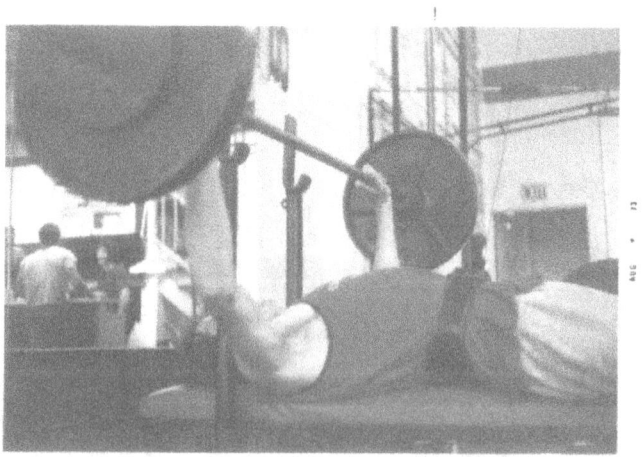

Benching at Gold's. Al Malone photo.

So when practicing the katas, at the moment of impact,

where you were executing a punch, all the muscles would be tensed.

I always kept my weight training a secret because of all the negative comments I would get about weight training at the dojo. I found that I was getting more flexible and faster as I practiced.

One thing though. For me, an ectomorph, it was very difficult to put on any muscle size. Yet I was extremely cut. And I was learning to move in ways I had never dreamed I could ever move before. As a youth I had been uncoordinated, clumsy. Now I could move in complicated patterns due to the practice of kata! And the weights in no way hindered me. I had found, at the time, the perfect solution to combining weight training and martial arts.

But there was still much more I was to learn.

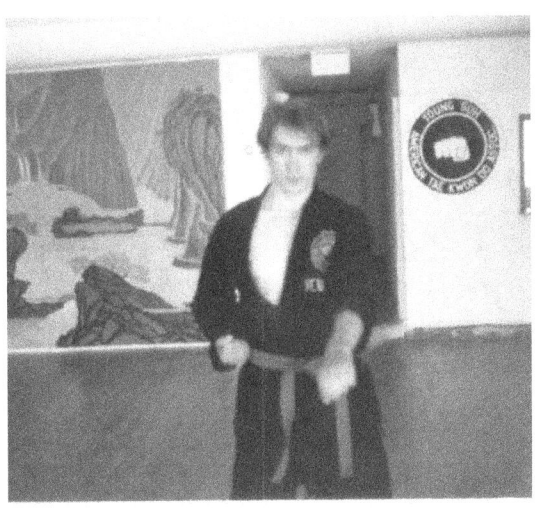

Practicing kata at Young Suh's in Burbank.
Al Malone photo.

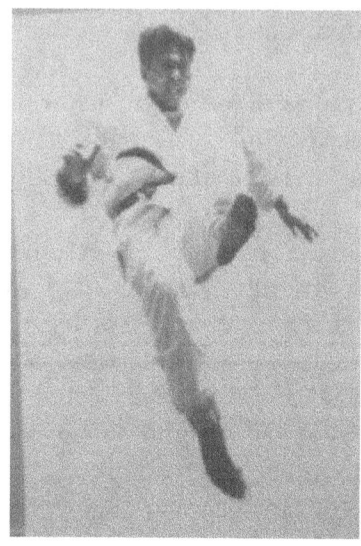

Master Young Suh, eighth degree black belt.

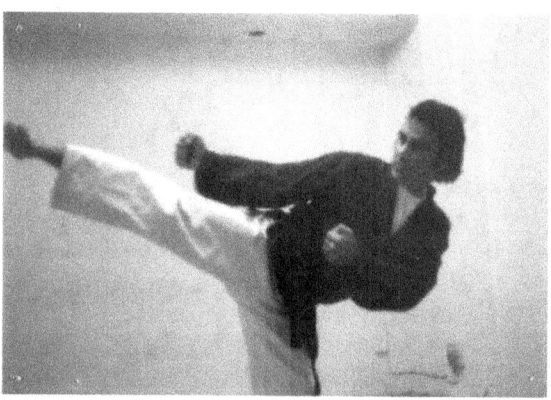

*Louie Vega, one of Young Suh's top instructors and my
teacher in taekwondo.*

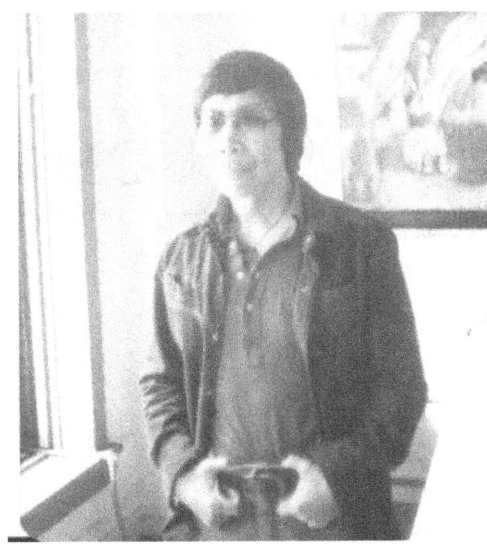

Sifu E.Y. Lee, kung fu master and former Mr. Chinatown, San Francisco.

CHAPTER ELEVEN
"THE INSTRUCTOR'S COURSE"

In the spring of 1975 I was doing my regular three times a week workouts. I was also training in martial arts at my sensei, Gus Johnson's school. One afternoon after work I went up to his garage dojo in San Rafael for the class but found that he had a barbecue party going on in his back yard.

Over beers and burgers he outlined to all of us that he was planning on holding a special instructor's course, to train certain select students to be instructors who would go to the local high schools and teach martial arts. He outlined his program.

There would be no charge for these classes. And when we became qualified instructors we would be paid as martial arts teachers. I was excited about this. At the time I was working at an apartment complex cleaning apartments and also doing grounds maintenance. It was a hard job, I had to go at a very fast pace. Then to my back room gym or to the dojo. I was able to do this because I practiced meditation. I will discuss more about this in another chapter.

Sensei outlined to us the way the course would be taught. It was to be extremely challenging. Three consecutive days in a row, Tuesday, Wednesday and Thursday evenings for three hours. It would be the hardest workout we ever had.

I was concerned. What about my Wednesday workout? Would I lose muscle? That was a main concern. It was very hard to gain muscle and do martial arts anyway. To not have that mid week workout? Would my build that I had worked so hard for survive? And the three hours martial arts workouts! Would that also drain away my muscle mass? This doesn't sound like such a big deal to most people, but to me, who had to fight for every gain I could get, it was a main cause for concern.

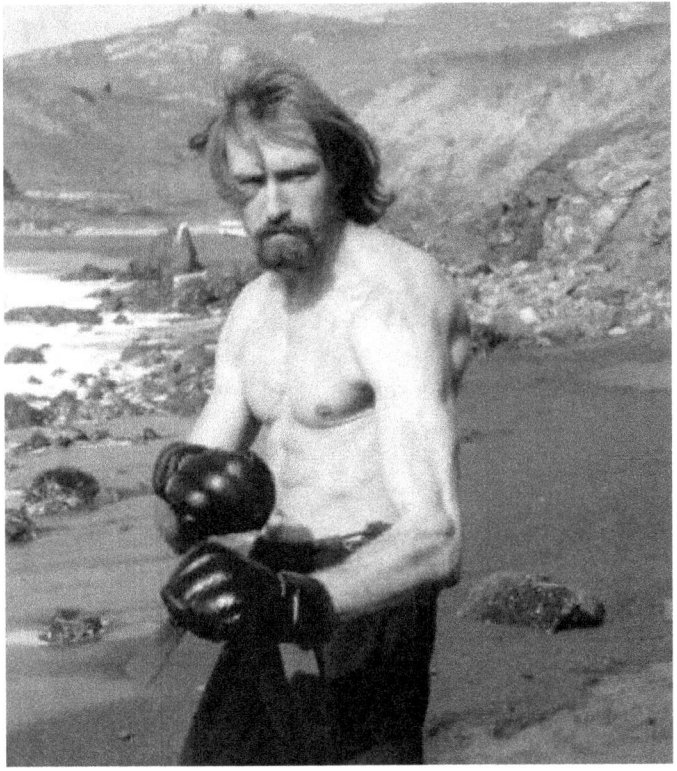

1977 at 30. Al Malone photo.

But, then I thought about what I would gain. I absolutely hated my day job. I was looking for a way out. To become a martial arts instructor and be paid for it? It sounded like a dream come true.

So I accepted the challenge.

Brief But Effective

I decided I would do a brief, abbreviated workout on Monday and Friday. I would work heavy and brief. And on Tuesday, Wednesday and Thursday I would go to the training course.

So I planned my workout strategy. My Monday workout looked like this:

Bench Press, ascending sets of three or two rep sets

Squats, one set of twenty reps

Pullups behind the neck, three sets of eight

Dumbell Curls, three sets of eight

Dips off bench, three sets of eight

I did full intensity on each and every set.

My Friday workout was a little bit different.

Bench Press, ascending sets of three or two reps sets, up to five sets

Deadlifts, ascending sets of two reps for up to five sets

Dumbbell Curls, three sets of eight

Dips off Bench, three sets of eight

Again, I did no ab work on this program. There were plenty of situps and leg raises in the intense martial arts workout.

The martial arts course was one of the most intense experiences I have ever had. Three hours of grueling hard work. We would stand in the deep horse stance for up to an hour doing blocking and punching drills. It was exhausting, it drained me of every ounce of energy. Plus I had to work my full time job.

At first I was pretty wasted and my weight training suffered. But, I got used to the schedule and pretty soon I actually saw a strength gain! It worked! Twice a week on an abbreviated routine worked!

It was a few months later that I became my sensei's weight training instructor.

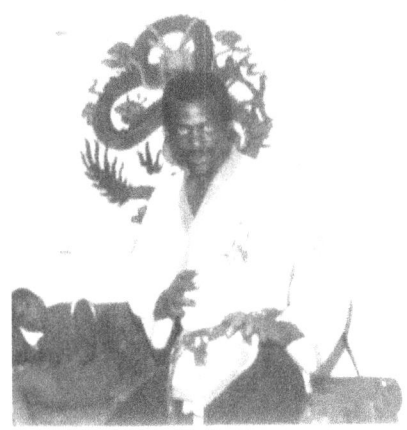

Grand Master Gus Johnson, 7ᵗʰ degree black belt.

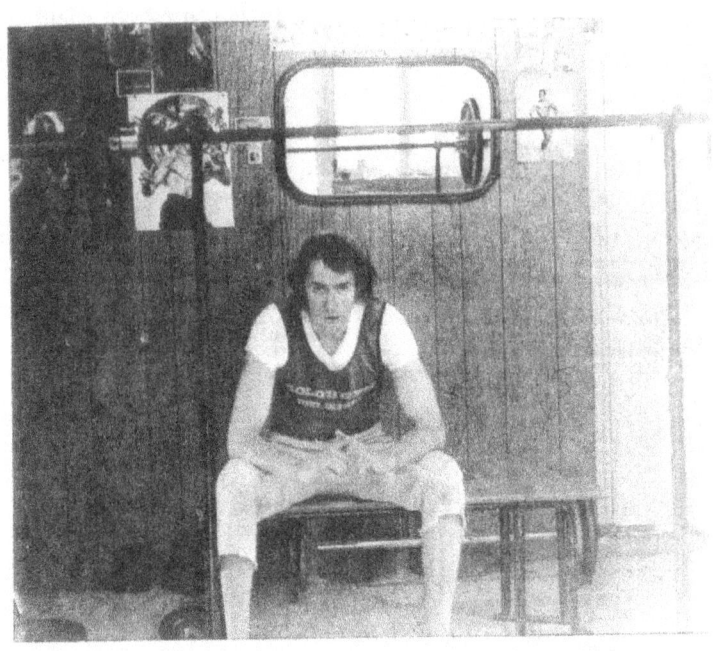

My backroom gym, 1975. Al Malone photo.

CHAPTER TWELVE, "MY OWN GYM"

I never got to finish the instructor's course. I had a severe bout of asthma which really knocked me down. I was really laid up although I was able to weight train to some extent. I called my sensei and told him I was going to have to drop out of the program. He told me I was welcome back any time. I thanked him and went about recovering, which was slow. This was in late 1975. By December I was well again and working out full steam at my back room gym, twice a week at a more extensive routine and also, I was training a few clients. One of my main students was Gene Orro, as I have said before, he was Sensei's top student and I trained him on the weights in secret as Sensei didn't really approve of weight training. I had utmost respect for Sensei but I firmly believed that weight training had only positive benefits. I strongly disagreed with the notion that weight training made one muscle bound or slowed them down. Gene Orro was the shining example of that.

So I was greatly surprised when Sensei showed up at my back room gym and said he had moved his school to a downtown location in San Rafael and that he wanted the new school to have a weight training instructor. I never asked how he found out that I trained people and he didn't tell me. He said I would have the entire back of the place as my own gym. He looked around at my basic equipment, Olympic barbell set, benches and regular iron barbells and dumbbells. He was highly impressed.

Thus, Pat Deu Pree's Gym was born in January of 1976. I

said good-by to that apartment complex job and set out on my new career, managing the dojo and my own gym.

During that time I had the opportunity to train over 200 students, personally, as well as my regular people who now came to my new gym to train. It was a fantastic time and I also really got deep into martial arts. I always divided up my training, back to three times a week on weights and three times a week on alternate days at martial arts. Because I didn't have a regular day job to suck my energy I was able to really absorb myself in my workouts. I had a pretty heavy schedule, sometimes training up to five people at a time. I learned to really manage my time.

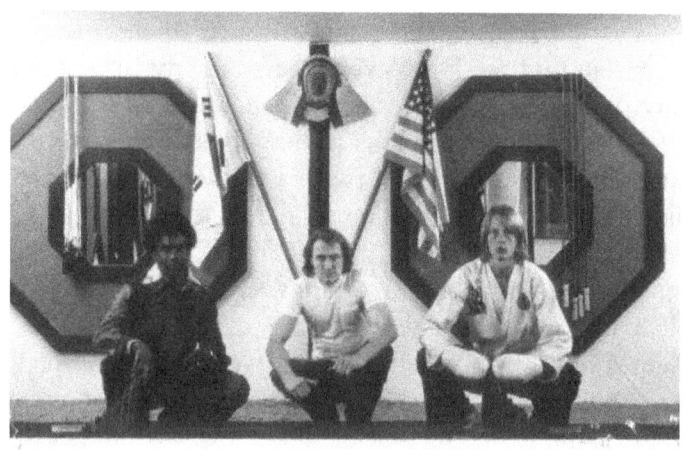

Two of my students, Michael, last name unknown , a boxer, to my right and to my left, Scott Jones.

Most of my students were also training at martial arts but I also had some hard core bodybuilding students. I learned much during that time about how to train others, putting to work all the thirteen years of weight training I had done.

I always taught the basics.

In 1977 the school moved to a new location, a larger building and at that time I met Dave Woodall. He was a young man who was a welder and also a motocross rider. He was a wild young man and really wanted to get into weight training. He looked around and said, "You need a lat machine."

Two days later he brought in a lat machine he had made in his father's welding shop. Two days later, a heavy duty bench he built. I paid him for the work and now I had extra equipment. During that time I hit on a new training strategy.

In *Muscular Development Magazine* I had read an article about a champion bodybuilder named Frank Calta. He was a top level competitor and also practiced martial arts. He had a new approach to training that I decided to try.

I never worked out on a split training routine. That is to say, a routine where you work certain body parts on one day and others on another day. That would have required me to work out at least four and up to six days a week. Being that I was doing martial arts on alternate days this was not possible. Thus, the rotating split routine.

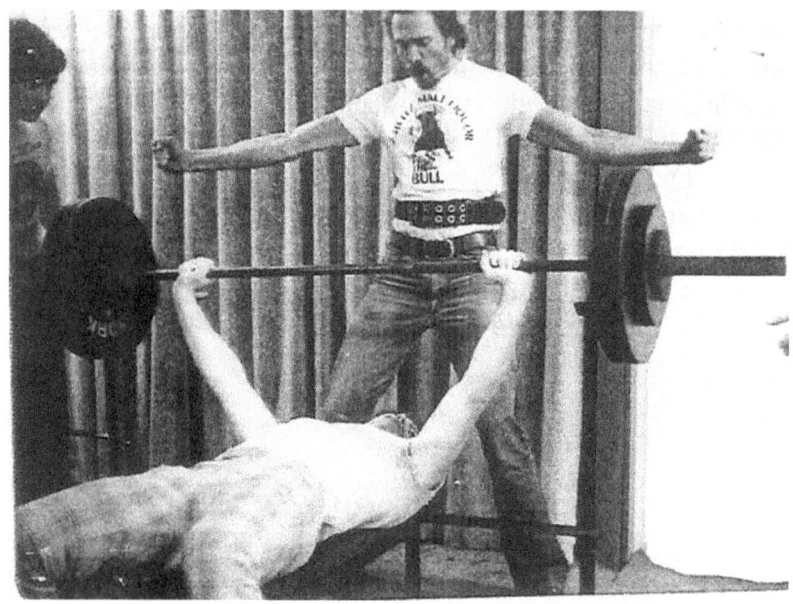

Spotting Mike O'Brien as he puts up 285 lbs.

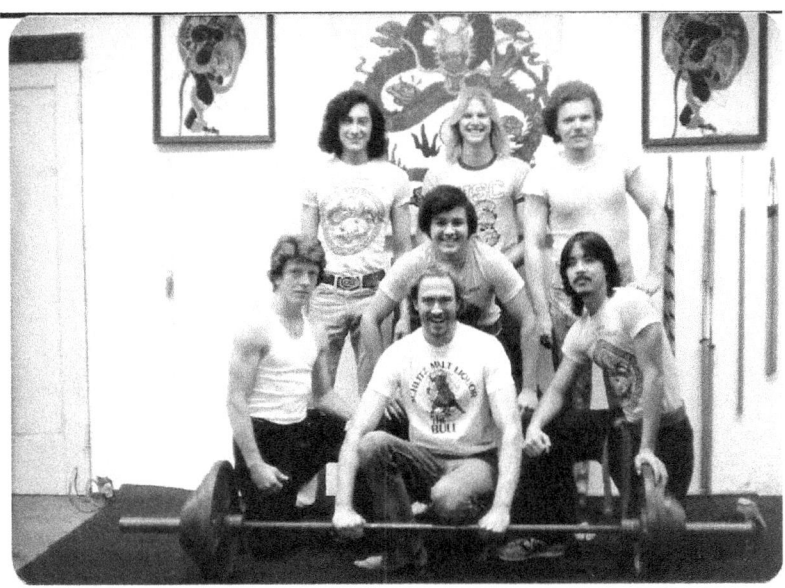

My chief members, 1978. Above left, John Cunningham, above middle, Dave Woodall, my equipment builder. Above right, Mike O'Brien. Center Kal Salama, to my left, Marcus Lee, on my right, unknown.

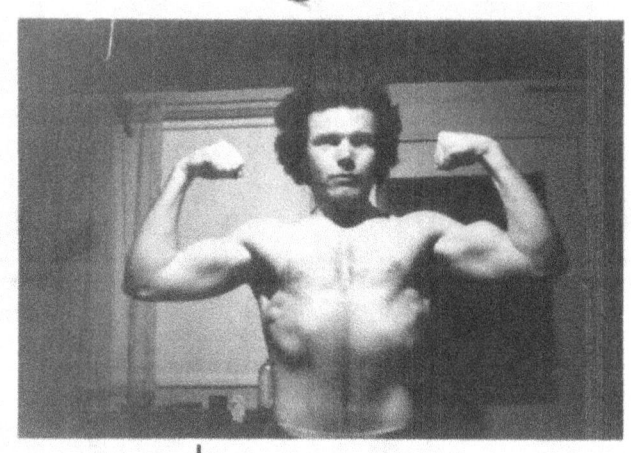

Mike O'Brien, fantastic natural bodybuilder.

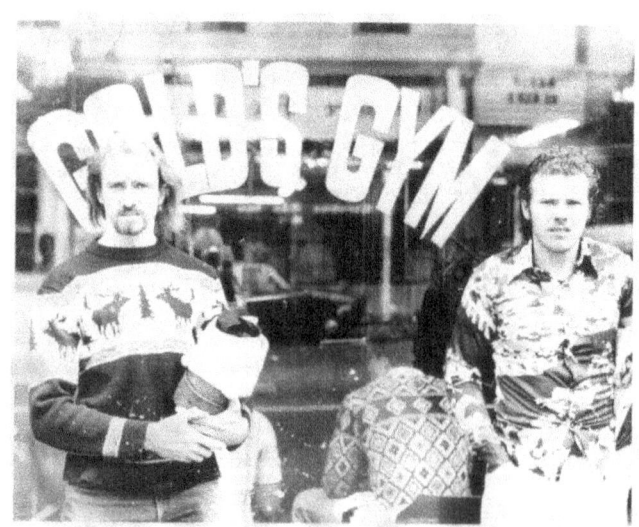

Me and Mike O'Brien at Gold's Gym in Santa Monica in 1978. Scott Gordon Photo.

CHAPTER THIRTEEN
"THE ROTATION SPLIT ROUTINE"

As I mentioned in the previous chapter, I read about the rotating split routine in *Muscular Development Magazine* in an article about a competitive bodybuilder named Frank Calta. He had come up with the idea of maximizing recovery. He felt that the usual six day a week split routine all bodybuilders were working out on was hindering his gains so he thought of trying something different. Thus, the rotating split routine was born.

I had always wanted to try a split routine but with karate on alternate days, it was just not possible. Now I had the answer! I immediately put all my weight training students on this routine.

The rotation routine works like this.

The first week, week 1, routine A. you work chest, shoulders and triceps on Monday and Friday. On Wednesday, routine B. legs, back and biceps are worked. On week 2, legs, back and biceps are worked on Monday and Friday. And on Wednesday of week 2, chest, shoulders and triceps are worked. Get the idea? And you rotate the routine from week to week, alternating routine A. and routine B.

This routine still enabled me to workout on martial arts on Tuesday, Thursday and Saturday and I had plenty of energy. I was still into high volume training at that time. I thought it was the most effective way to train. I was, in later years, to find a better way but that is for a future chapter.

I immediately saw improvement. I was able to do a variety of exercises for each body part. As usual, for me, ab work was done on the days that I practiced martial arts. This is what the rotating workout looked like:

Workout A

Bench Press	4x8-10
Incline Bench Press	4x8-10
Seated Behind the Neck Press	4x8-10
Dumbbell Lateral Raises	4x8-10
Lying Triceps Extension	4x8-10
Triceps Pushdown on Lat Machine	4x8-10

Workout B

Squats	4x8-10
Heel Raises	4x15
Dead Hang Power Cleans	4x8-10
Behind Neck Lat Pulldowns	4x8-10
Pulldowns to Chest	4x8-10
Barbell Curls	4x8-10
Dumbbell Curls	4x8-10

I finally had a lat machine so I put it to good use. To note, I do not recommend either the seated press behind the neck or the lat pulldown behind the neck anymore. It's too damaging to the rotator cuff. The last year I practiced behind the neck presses was when I was 55 and I got seriously injured as a result.

I have included the dead hand power clean here. It is a fantastic growing exercise for the whole body. Although I was not able to continue this exercise in my fifties I recommend it. I just can't do that exercise anymore due to hip injuries.

The dead hand power clean:

Squat down and take hold of the barbell. Take a deep breath. With a heave, using the momentum of your entire body, clean the weight up until it rests at shoulder level in front of you. Now, lower the weight to hang at your thighs. Using the momentum of your entire body clean the weight back up to shoulder level. I recommend you ask a personal trainer about this one. This is an exercise used by football players for overall body power. The reason I discontinued this exercise is because it began tearing my hip muscles after I was 54 years of age. It was one of my favorite power exercises. But due to age and my personal physical problems, for me, I could no longer continue this exercise. I use the stiff legged deadlift instead.

The rotation split routine enables one to work out on a split routine and yet, maximize recovery. This can be used not only for martial arts, but also any sport you might be pursuing. Rock climbing, tennis, etc. Train on weights on certain days and practice your sport on the alternate day. Or, if you are into building mass, then simply rest on the alternate day. The alternate day can also be used to perform aerobic exercise such as running and cycling. The alternating split routine is a great way to train if you like high volume.

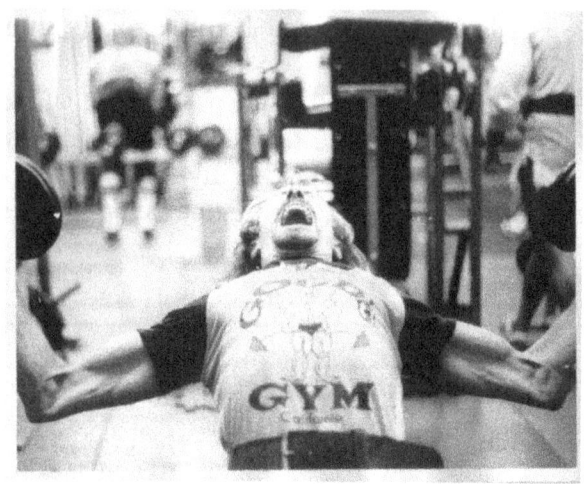

Just how hard can a set be? Scott Gordon Photo

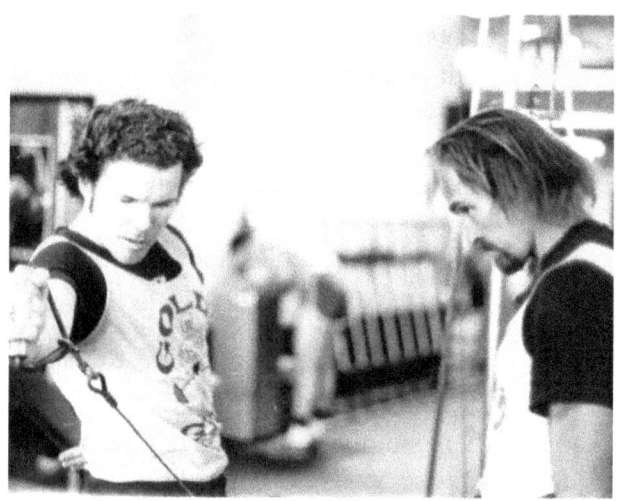

*Coaching Mike O'Brien on the finer points. Scott Gordon
Photo.*

CHAPTER FOURTEEN
"RECOVERY"

I am going to talk more about recovery in this chapter. Recovery is the name of the game in strength training. Especially so in heavy weight training routines. If you train every day at high volume you can run the risk of overtraining. Too many sets and reps, not enough recovery days can lead to fatigue and chronic injuries. I've been down that road before.

In 1982 I was training with a training partner. I had taught him the rotating split routine. We began training longer and longer, adding more sets. We were training at an insane pace. Even though we were using the rotating split routine it was still too much. Especially for me. A hard gainer. And I had just turned 35. That's when I began to notice something. The recovery curve was getting longer.

You hear every day in the news about sports stars who are getting into their late thirties constantly getting injured. It becomes chronic. That is because, even though in your thirties you can still train extremely hard or play extremely hard, the body just doesn't recover quickly enough.

I began doing more and more sets and found that with some workouts, I had endless energy, but on others, my warm up seemed heavy. By elbows began hurting, I was developing chronic tendonitis. I would go to the gym three times a week and train for up to two hours. Using the rotation program I should have been more rested. But now I was mid thirties. My body had changed.

Not only were my elbows in constant pain, but my

hamstrings were also constantly sore. And something else was happening as well. I began to lose muscle size and gain fat!

I had to rethink my strategy. I went back to every thing I had read in the bodybuilding magazines before. I found the answer in the old *Iron Man* magazines, the ones that were published by the original publisher, Peary Rader. I read articles by Arthur Jones, the originator of the Nautilus machines and training system. By his protégé, Mike Mentzer and his brother Ray. Articles by Stuart McRobert and Bradley J. Steiner. They all recommended briefer, less frequent routines.

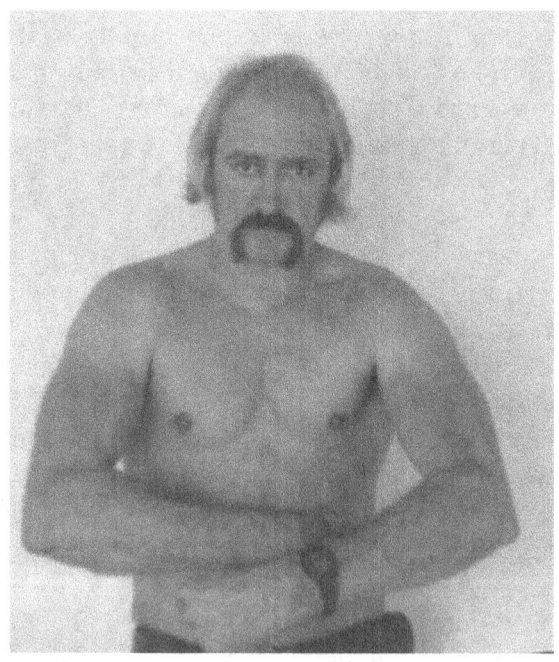

Gaining mass is all about recovery. Photo, Amanda Torres.

I decided to completely change my training.

I had stopped training with my training partner by then and was going it alone, as I usually do. I was working out at a very hard core bodybuilding gym at the time, the Astro Gym, down in San Gabriel Valley in southern California. And I would also go out to Gold's Gym in Venice from time to time.

I decided I would only train twice a week. Light on Wednesday and heavy on Saturday mornings. I would do only three sets for bench press and squats and only two sets for lat pulls, presses behind the neck and for curls and triceps extensions.

A fantastic thing happened! I dropped fat and put on an extra twenty pounds of solid muscle. This was at the age of 37 in the summer of 1984. I had also added amino acids. More about amino acids later.

Everyone who saw me was highly impressed. I was actually bigger than when I was 25 when I had been training for three hours a day three days a week. Now my workouts only lasted about an hour and a quarter. A bit longer on Saturday mornings because I would do lower reps and more sets on the bench press working up to doubles and singles, more of a power lifting workout.

I want to make a point here that all this time I was working at a full time job that was physically demanding. And yet, I had just made the greatest gains of my life.

Like I said, the name of the game is recovery. I had the needed rest and I grew.

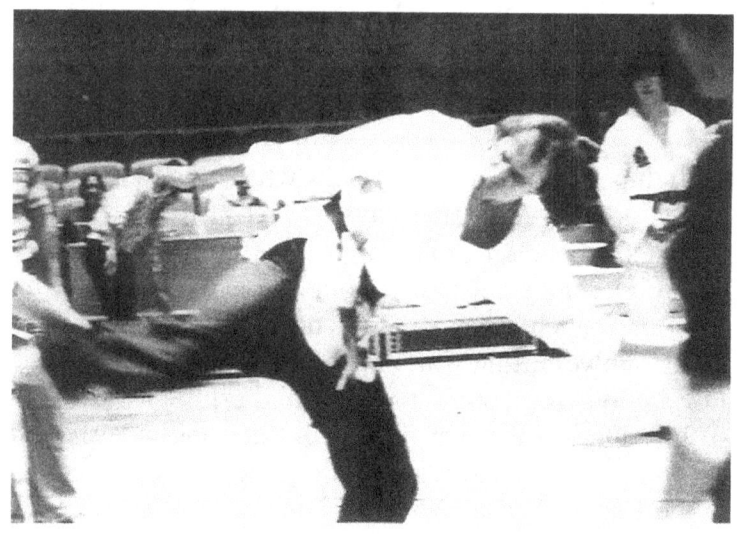

The Oakland Arena, 1977.

CHAPTER FIFTEEN
"CARDIO"

I am not a big fan of cardiovascular exercise. It saps needed energy for muscle gains, it also can deplete muscle size. I did cardio mostly in the form of jumping rope back during my martial arts years. These were not years where I had a lot of muscle mass, I was, however, really "cut". I had the "Bruce Lee" look.

Nevertheless, cardio is important. It's just that it has been highly overrated.

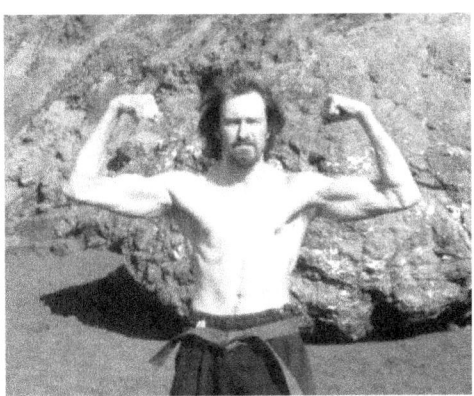

Cardio is any exercise that works the heart and lungs for an extended period of time. Most recommendations are at least 45 minutes of cardio a day. I do not agree with this, I do not believe it's necessary. Unless, that is, you are training for a marathon. Then you are specializing. You'll notice that top marathon runners do not have a lot of muscle mass on their bodies.

Too much cardio can compromise the immune system and deplete testosterone! A needed element in well being and building muscle mass.

When I practiced martial arts I would jump rope for a half hour before my workout. The martial arts routine itself was a total cardio workout. I was in great shape but I was frustrated. I wanted more muscle mass and on weight training days I worked out hard and heavy, but I just could not put on much size. I accepted this at that time because I was specializing in martial arts.

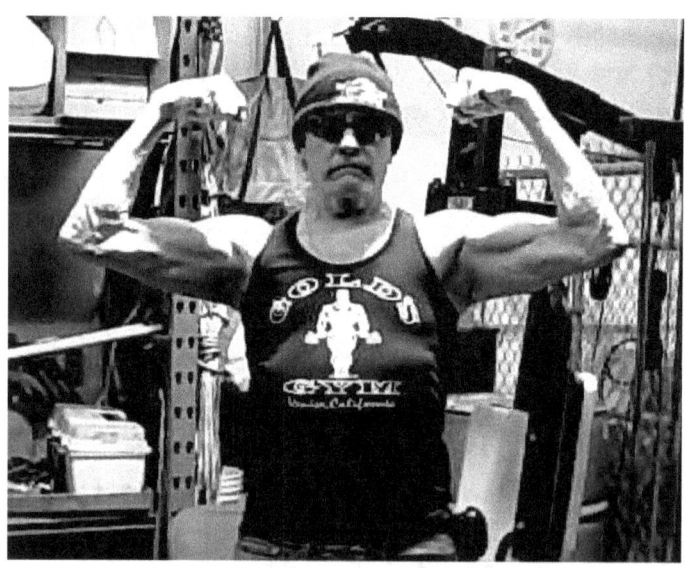

At 65. Properly trained muscles can last a lifetime.

In my fifties and into my early sixties I would ride my bicycle to work, it was only four miles and I was in great shape cardio wise. And I did my usual once a week basic workout with the weights. The bike ride took only twenty minutes and did not sap my energy. In fact, on the ride home on my workout day, it was a good warm-up. I don't ride anymore. I like to take walks, which is also a great overall fitness exercise. Too much stress is placed on hard cardio workouts as the only way to keep fit. This is not true. Overall, one can keep in great shape by just taking long walks. If you are interested in gaining muscle size, then specialize on just weight training for a period of time until you have gained a good level of size and strength. At that point then adding some cardio can help you get "cut". A certain amount of cardio will help burn body fat.

Just weight training alone will burn body fat as the body builds muscle. This is done during the period of rest between weight training workouts. As the body recovers it automatically burns fat as muscle is being built.

So be careful as to the amount of cardio you perform.

CHAPTER SIXTEEN
"WOMEN AND WEIGHT TRAINING"

Can women benefit from weight training?

They most certainly can. Both women and men can benefit greatly from strength training using weights. In fact, weight training should be an important part of a women's fitness routine. Weight training not only builds muscle but it also, as I have previously said, builds strong bones. As women age their muscles deteriorate causing them to have hip fractures and a bent spine. You've seen the "horseshoe" spine elderly women have? It comes from having weak muscles. As muscle is built, so is bone.

Some common misconceptions about weight training women have is that they will put on "too much muscle".

I have heard women tell me, "But I don't want muscles."

Yes, you do want muscles. In fact, without muscles you couldn't breathe, walk, digest food, talk, etc.

The fear is that the moment they touch a weight they will automatically look like a massive, competitive bodybuilder. Nothing is further than the truth. For one thing, it's almost impossible for most people, men or women, to build such mass.

Women produce less testosterone than men do so they will never be able to gain as much muscle as a man can.

What about competitive women bodybuilders?

These are women who are elite athletes, they have a superior genetic advantage when it comes to building muscles and they work full time at it. Women who adopt the basic weight training routines I have outlined twice a week, or even once a week, will build strength that will benefit all areas of their lives. So I strongly recommend that women add strength training to their fitness routine.

Performing two sets of eight to ten repetitions of the following routine is all you really need to build useful, functional strength.

Bench Press

Squats

Dumbbell Rows

Dumbbell Seated Press

Curls

Lying Triceps Extensions

This simple routine can be done once or twice a week for great results. You will notice body fat burned and a more "toned" athletic look. You will be able to move easier, household chores will become a breeze, you will have a greater feeling of well being.

I trained a women once who was making great progress. Her entire body was looking different, sleek, toned and she felt great. Then one day she said to me, "Yes, but I haven't lost any weight."

Don't let the scale dictate your life! Muscle weighs more than fat so you may not see yourself losing a lot of weight, but your body composition will change completely.

I once said to a woman who had put on ten pounds of healthy muscle and burned fat, "What would an added ten pounds of muscle feel like if you found yourself alone in a parking lot at night?"

I always recommend that women take a self defense course. Women should be able to defend themselves, and there is nothing wrong with a woman being strong!

To be bone thin is not healthy. The entertainment and fashion world places unreal demands on women to look a certain way and it destroys their lives. Bone thin is not good for your bone structure as you get older. That bent back look and hip fractures are the results of such extremes.

A women once asked me, "Pat, what do you think of five pound weights?"

"I think that's pure bullshit," was my answer!

Five pound weights are a good workout for a two year old but not for long. Doing endless repetitions with five pound dumbbells is useless.

Challenge yourself!

If you can do more than twelve repetitions with a weight, then use a heavier weight. A rule of thumb here is to stay in the range of about six to twelve repetitions. If you can't do six in proper form, it's too heavy. If you can get more than twelve, it's time to add about five to ten pounds.

Weight training is a valuable addition to any woman's strength training routine and I highly recommend it.

CHAPTER SEVENTEEN
"THE ONE BODYPART A DAY ROUTINE"

Bodybuilders today have changed their way of training, due the impact of Mike Mentzer, Arthur Jones and others who got them thinking on a slightly different track. When I pick up a copy of a bodybuilding magazine I have noticed that bodybuilders are using briefer routines then before and many have adopted the one bodypart a day routine. They work each bodypart once a week but workout five or six days a week.

I usually never advocate six day a week training. But sometimes I see that some trainers need to workout every day.

A friend told me he had bought an entire home gym setup but that he never seemed to have time to train. "I just don't have the time, what with kids and work and other responsibilities."

I thought about it for a moment. I was going to advise him to follow a once a week basic routine but something told me not to suggest that. He had good genetics, a natural for bodybuilding. He would not easily fall into an overtraining rut. So I told him, his name was Jonny, "Jonny, tell you what. The minute you get home from work, run out into that garage before you do anything else and just hit one exercise. For instance, on Monday, go out and just do bench presses. Then Tuesday, do squats, Wednesday, lat machine, Thursday, seated press, Friday, curls, and Saturday, Triceps. Got the idea?"

He thought about it and it's like a lightbulb went off in his brain. So he gave it a try. He told me it was working very well. He had put on muscle mass and always had time to do the brief one exercise a day routine.

Then one day I noticed he was avoiding me. I didn't think much about it at the time until I asked him how the routine was coming along.

"Well, to tell you the truth, Pat, one day I decided to do some laundry first before training and then I ended up never going back. There just seemed to be too many things to do suddenly."

One missed workout and it had all fallen apart. Though I don't recommend every day training I know that for some people, if they don't hit it every day then they simply stop training. So for many, training every day is exactly what they need. And if you are not a "hard gainer" then it won't stop your progress.

The reason I advocate less frequency is because, for hard gainers, more rest is needed in order for the body to recover and grow.

Another friend of mine, his name is Al, works out on a similar program. It seems to work for him. Here is an example of a brief one exercise a day routine:

Monday: Bench Press	4x6-8
Tuesday: Squats	4x6-8
Wednesday: Rows	4x6-8
Thursday: Standing Press	4x6-8
Friday: Curls	4x6-8
Saturday: Triceps Ext.	4x6-8
Sunday: Rest	

Each workout lasts about ten minutes. Each set is worked hard. Al is a natural, puts on muscle size easily, so this works very well for him.

I have read articles about bodybuilders in their fifties and sixties and even seventies who have adopted similar routines, although they do more exercises for each bodypart, but they have found that training each bodypart once a week enables them to train hard and not overtrain.

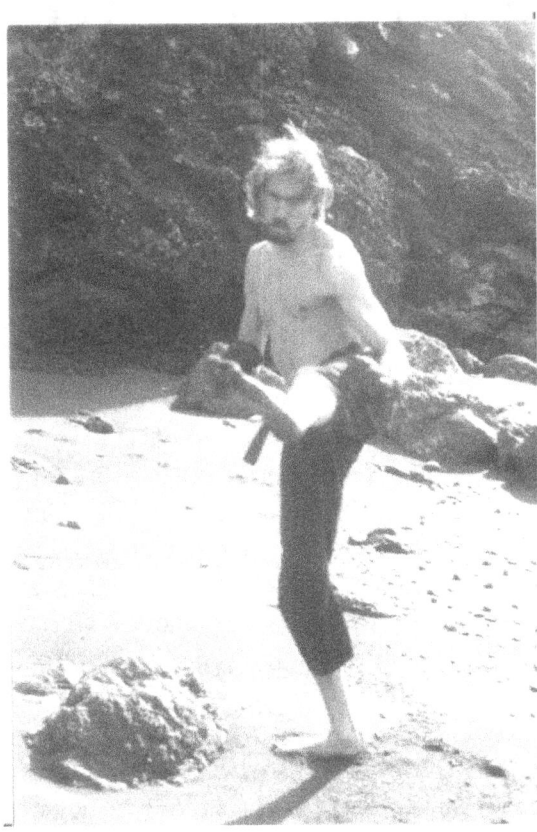

CHAPTER EIGHTEEN
"THE TWICE A WEEK HIGH VOLUME SPLIT"

Back in 2008 I was attending night classes at Glendale College. They have a really fantastic weight room there, power cages, Olympic barbell sets, heavy duty benches, everything for a really hard core basic workout.

In earlier years, sometimes before class I would sneak into the weight room and take a brief basic workout. The usual, bench presses, squats, lat pulls, presses, curls triceps extensions. Then I would go to my usual class. But as the years went on the security got tighter and tighter at the weight room. One of the football coaches knew I worked out there and it was fine with him, watching me work out he knew that I knew what I was doing. I would even sometimes give training tips to some of the younger guys.

Finally, they got a system where you had to swipe an ID card at the front desk to get in and there was no way around it. So I stopped working out there completely. Things had changed. They had another workout room upstairs but that was mostly cardio and machines. When I inquired about working out they told me I could use the room upstairs or the heavy duty weight room downstairs. Guess which one I chose?

So I decided to sign up for a semester. You actually got a credit for working out there. But, there was a catch. Always is, right?

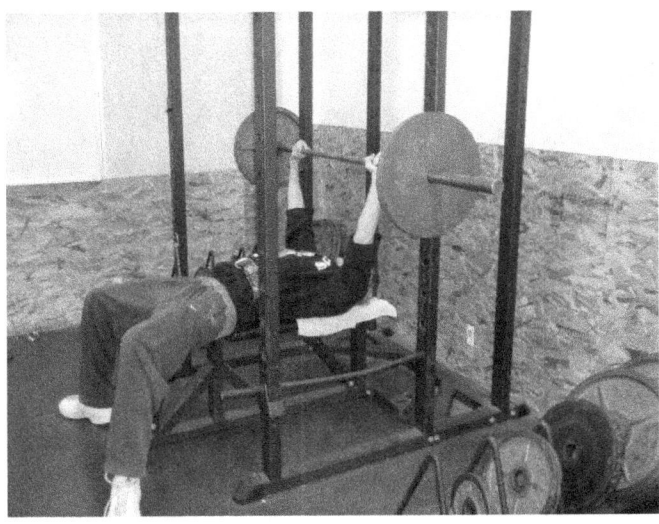

Bench pressing in the power cage at Glendale College weight room.

You had to put in a certain amount of time and it was logged in based on the swipe of your card both going in and leaving the weight room. To get the credit you had to work out a certain amount of hours. I decided on a two day a week workout. I realized that I would have to work out at least two hours per workout to get the amount of time required. After the time had been accumulated then I could lower the volume of training.

So I thought about it. It was a challenge. Plus, I realized that amount of time working out was not needed. But few realize the high intensity principle I have been promoting for the past thirty years or so.

I decided to do a two day split. I would work out on Tuesday and Thursday. I would split the routine up, upper body on Tuesday and lower body on Thursday and I would hit it for two hours. I figured working each body part once a week would give me plenty of days to recover.

My workout looked something like this:

Tuesday

Bench Press, ascending five or two rep sets for a total of five to seven sets.
Dumbbell Incline, five sets of eight.
Pec Deck, five sets of ten.
Military Presses on machine, five sets of eight
Alternating Dumbbell Seated Presses, five sets of eight
Barbell Curls, five sets of eight
Lying Triceps Extensions, five sets of eight
Dumbbell Curls, five sets of ten
Triceps Pushdowns on Lat Machine, five sets of ten.
Also, before the workout, twenty five ab crunches on lat machine and twenty five leg lifts on the captain's chair for lower abs.

On Thursday the workout looked like this:

Ab work to warm up as described above.
Squats in Power Cage, five to seven sets of ascending sets of five reps.
Thigh Extensions on machine, five sets of ten reps.
Thigh Curls on machine, five sets of ten reps.
Leg Presses on machine, five sets of ten reps.
Stiff legged deadlifts, one set of ten.
Shrugs on Machine, five sets of eight.
Four Way Free Hand Neck Exercise, two sets of twenty each way.
Forearm Curls, two sets of twenty.
Reverse Forearm Curls, two sets of twenty.

That was the routine. Lots of volume, much more than I usually recommend. But with the extra rest days, I found I had high energy! Before leaving the house for each workout I would have a protein drink consisting of two cups of non fat lactose free milk, two scoops of egg protein and a banana. And, in the locker room, just before the workout I would have a protein bar. I carried a plastic bottle of water with me to sip during the grueling workout.

I absolutely loved it! In a hard core basic workout room with all the weights at my command! And I was getting a college credit as well! I couldn't have been happier. I found that I was gaining in strength and energy. And that was at the age of 61!

I was able to do high volume and with all the rest days in between I was able to maximize recovery.

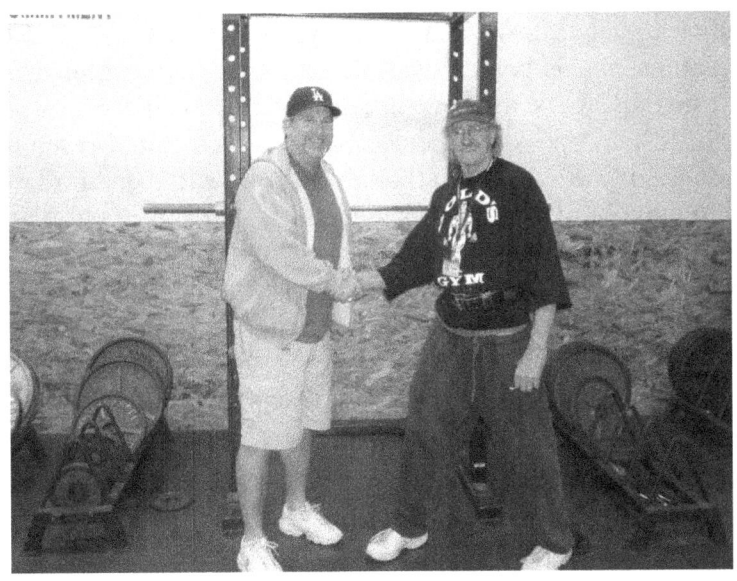

Coach meets coach at Glendale College weight room.

CHAPTER NINETEEN
"BUILDING MASS"

Now I am going to talk about building mass. Muscle size, gaining solid weight.

If you are really skinny and weak there is an answer. I know, I walked down that road myself. As I have said at the beginning of this book, I was an extreme case, weighing only 120 pounds at six foot one and a half! You can see from the pictures, they speak for themselves. And you can also see that I was highly successful although it took years because I was finding out how my body responded.

If you are too thin and weak then you are going to want to specialize for at least a year to gain healthy weight. During that time I suggest that you do no cardiovascular workouts at all. No running, no cycling, no other athletic activity. You want to concentrate completely on gaining muscle size and any other activity will sap your recovery ability.

For the workout, you will do the basic routine I have already outlined earlier. I will now refresh your memory.

Ab crunches, 25
Leg lifts off bench, 25

Bench Press	2x7
Squats	1x20
Bent Row or	
Dumbbell Row	2x7
Standing Press	2x7

| Curls | 2x7 |
| Lying Triceps Ext | 2x7 |

Do this workout twice a week with at least two days in between. For example, Monday and Thursday, or Tuesday and Friday, or Wednesday and Saturday. Make sure you get enough rest in between and get at least eight hours of sleep at night.

Now I want to talk a bit about the twenty rep squat mentioned above. This is the absolute key to the program. Squats, as I have mentioned before, are the chief gaining exercise for the entire body. There is a way to do this exercise. It is the most intense experience you will ever have. Monte Hargraves, my main training partner of the past twenty five years will attest to that.

Back in 1992 we worked out at a hard core gym in Burbank called The Power Source. Many top bodybuilders worked out there as well as some of the champion pro wrestlers of the day. Wayne Coleman, known as Superstar Billy Graham and other notables in the pro wrestling world.

One day Monte and I were over at the squat rack. I asked him if he wanted to try the twenty rep squat. He said, "Yeah, sure." He didn't know what he was in for.

This is how you do it.

Take the weight from the rack resting on the back of the shoulders, not the back of the neck. Walk out from the rack and stand with feet shoulder width apart. Take a deep breath and squat down, letting the air explode out of your lungs as you drive back up to the starting position. Do this for ten reps. By now you should be really tired. But you're not done yet! Now, rest a moment and take in two breaths before descending. Do three more reps with two breaths between each rep. That's 13 reps now. But you're not done yet. And you are feeling really wasted! But it isn't over yet. Now, take three or four breaths before descending! That's right, keep going. Do three more reps this way, that's 16 reps done! Only four more to go! You feel like you're dying, right? But it isn't over. Now take five to six breaths and do the last four this way. Then rack the weight! You should feel like you have just run into a brick wall!

After doing the twenty rep set as described Monte fell to the floor. He looked like he had had a religious experience! He had never, ever worked so hard.

So that is how you do the twenty rep set of squats. And you only need one set. I don't think you even want to contemplate another set!

Get the idea?

This is how solid muscle gains are made over your entire body!

A word about doing squats. Never pad the bar. Some trainers put a pad or a towel around the bar. You don't need to do that, it makes the bar unstable. If you ride the bar low across the back of your shoulders you will find you do not need a pad. I have seen men squat 600 lbs without a pad.

Monte and I were at the Power Source gym one afternoon. We approached the squat rack. There was a foam pad on the bar. Monte took the pad off and said, "We sure don't need this **&&$ thing!" He gave it a toss and it was last seen flying ceiling high across that massive warehouse sized gym to actually land at a squat rack all the way on the other side of the gym!

Don't pad the bar. Monte just may be watching!

The Secret to Gains!

Now for the secret to fantastic gains. GOMAD!

What is GOMAD? It's the secret to gaining solid mass in the shortest time that nature will allow. GOMAD means, a gallon of milk a day!

That's right, a gallon of milk a day. To gain muscle mass you need plenty of the right kind of protein and especially enough calories. There is really no other way to gain a great deal of muscle size. You have to rest enough and you have to eat enough food to maintain yourself and to gain extra muscle.

This is usually the place where you ask, "What about my cuts?"

Look, Pal, you're skinny as a rail, no appreciable muscle on you whatsoever! Forget about being "cut" for now. You need muscle on your frame and lots of it! Once you have gained all the size you can gain in a year then worry about refining it. You have to have the "clay" to mold your physique with. Stick to this basic routine.

Now, in addition to drinking a gallon of milk a day I want you to also add a level cup of whey protein to the mix. Break the gallon of milk with protein powder up into many servings and drink it down during the day. Take it to work with you in a plastic bottle in an ice chest or in a thermos bottle.

You want to also eat plenty of protein rich foods. The following is an example of the mass gaining diet:

Breakfast: Four eggs, lean ground beef, toast, coffee, a piece of fruit and a protein drink.

Mid morning: Protein drink.

Lunch: Two meat and cheese sandwiches, two pieces of fruit and a protein drink.

Mid afternoon: Protein drink. And on workout day, a protein drink before your workout.

Dinner: Meat, potatoes or natural brown rice, a fresh steamed vegetable and a protein drink.

Just before bed: Protein drink.

This program should find you many solid pounds heavier at the end of a year. You have to give it a year, there is no such thing as instant muscles. Building solid muscle mass takes time, it's not an overnight thing and any advertisement that tells you different is a fraud! Believe me, I've been there. It just doesn't work.

After a year assess your progress. If you are very much improved, have built a lot of mass in that time, you just may be someone who could give professional bodybuilding a shot. Only time will tell. Otherwise, by all means continue to work out, just realize that you don't have the genetics for great muscle mass. That was a mistake I made and it was very costly. It cost me my education in my youth and thus many opportunities I could have had. It was many years later that I got the message and went to school, and with the knowledge that I actually needed only a very intense, brief, basic routine once a week, I kept the gains I had made in muscle and also created other opportunities as well.

Amino Acids

I mentioned amino acids before and I want to talk about them now. Amino acids are a great way to help create muscle mass, especially if you're over 35. I had my first experience with amino acids back in 1984 at 37 when I was working out at the Astro Gym in San Gabriel Valley. As I said before, I had made the greatest gains of my life that summer. And amino acids helped me gain the muscle size. Lou Greenburg, the owner of the Astro Gym, handed me a bottle of Unipro Free Form and Peptide Bond Amino Acids and said, "Try one bottle and if you don't see results then you never have to buy another bottle."

So I tried them and wow! What a difference. I had enhanced energy and added muscle growth!

Let me explain for a moment about the difference between amino acids and steroids. Steroids are testosterone which bodybuilders use to enhance muscle gains. This is putting added testosterone in the body which can, in time, cause the body to lose its natural ability to produce its own testosterone. There area cases of bodybuilders experiencing gynomastia, or breast growth as a result.

With amino acids, you help your own body produce its own testosterone and growth hormone which aids in muscle growth and a feeling of well being. Today I take 1000 milligrams of L-Arganine and I have experienced great results. I had noticed my chest had gone down even though I was working out hard. After adding the L-Arganine my chest and arm measurements returned to their original size. After 35 your body begins to produce less testosterone and growth hormone. Doing squats and deadlifts help the body to create more of its own. Amino acids help with this process. Be sure you buy free form and peptide bond amino acids as they are easily utilized by the body.

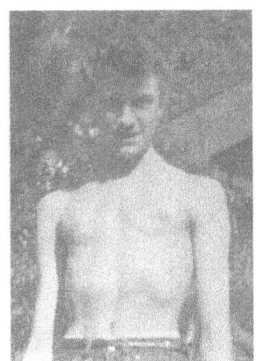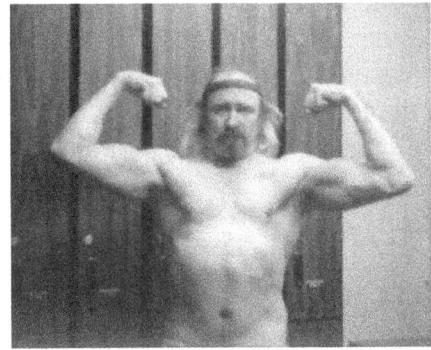

In my case, it took years. Knowing what I know now, it would have been a lot faster. The photo at the right was taken at the Power Source in 1992 on my 45th birthday.

CHAPTER TWENTY
"THE OTHER SIDE OF ACTION"

So far I have outlined ways you can work out to stay in shape for life. But there is the other side of the coin. Getting away from the action phase and into the deep, calm state where everything is regenerated.

For the past 47 years I have practiced Transcendental Meditation (TM) twice a day. I am not being paid to recommend this program by the Transcendental Meditation organization. I am sharing this because I have had profound benefits from meditating twice a day.

Meditating takes you to a deep level of restful awareness where you can regenerate your forces. It's like taking a bath in deep relaxation.

Mindfulness

A way anyone can meditate is this, and it doesn't take a lot of time, only about ten to fifteen minutes. It's called "mindfulness". Simply sit quietly and close your eyes. Become aware of your breathing, don't try to concentrate hard at it, just sit and be aware. As you do you will notice yourself going into a quieter, more relaxed state of mind. Thoughts will come and go, don't worry about them, just observe them. Don't force yourself. Then gently come out of the relaxed state, open your eyes and go about your daily tasks. You will find yourself more aligned with life, have more energy and you will just seem to get things done in an easier way. The results are cumulative over time. Meditation should be a part of everyone's program along with working out. It is the other side of the coin.

I've heard the excuses. "I just don't have time to meditate, I have too much to do now."

I have a friend who I taught how to meditate. He is one of the busiest people I have ever seen. I told him, "Just step away for ten minutes and give it a try." He did and told me, "Yeah, it worked, but, I lost ten minutes of work I could have been doing."

I had to walk away from that one. There is an old saying, "Don't push the river." When you meditate you cease "pushing the river" and you begin to flow with the current of life. You will find, no matter how busy you are, that things will just seem to get done without as much effort. This is something you have to experience, you may not notice it right away. I get up earlier just so I can get my meditation in because it sets up my day to face everything I have to face and things usually work themselves out.

I strongly recommend the Transcendental Meditation program but otherwise, at least try the mindful meditation method I have just described above. You will find benefits that will stay with you for your entire lifetime. It's worth it to take the extra time to meditate.

CHAPTER TWENTY ONE
"THE MYTH OF TONING AND LENGTHENING"

I have read various books and seen videos of exercise by so called experts. One thing that stands out clearly is the myth of toning and lengthening.

The myth of toning

First, there is no such thing as "toning" the muscles. You don't "tone" the muscles. You build them. Muscles are either being built or they are deteriorating. This doesn't mean that you are gaining muscles size all the time, but it means that the breakdown and build up of muscle tissue is always going on. If one has a slender look to their muscles then it is said that the muscles are "toned". And if someone has large muscles it is said that they are "bulky". Bulky, as if that's a bad thing. People seem to be absolutely terrified of having larger muscles! They avoid certain exercises because "experts" say that they will become "bulky".

I do a heavy basic routine that so called experts would say would automatically make me "bulky". It never happened. At least not to the extent I was trying to achieve. The larger muscles of a competition bodybuilder are highly efficient muscles. Just take a look at Jean Claude Van Damme. Extremely muscular, was a competitive bodybuilder in addition to being a fantastic martial artist. One only has to see how he moves in his movies. So muscles that are large are very useful when applied to other activities.

If you desire not to have bulky muscles, then just eat a moderate diet while you work out and you will stay at a certain level that you are happy with. My body has the look of a "toned" body, slender but muscular. Certain "experts" have said, "Oh, you obviously do a 'toning' routine."

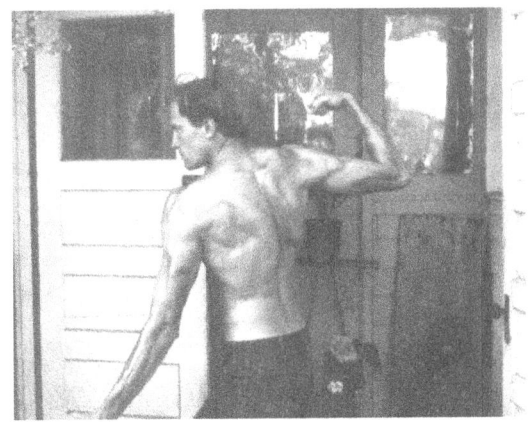

Well defined muscles are said to be "toned".

I do all the basic exercises, bench presses, squats, rows, deadlifts, etc. that would make a natural at this game very large and muscular and with adding more food and protein drinks I have been able to, at times, greatly add muscle size on my small boned frame. When I was highly involved in martial arts it was extremely hard to gain muscle size so I stayed at a certain level and concentrated on karate. But I always lifted weights.

The myth of lengthening

The next myth I want to talk about is the myth of lengthening the muscles.

Certain exercise experts, in fact a great number, say that

you can "lengthen" the muscles by doing certain routines and that by doing weight training you will "shorten" the muscles.

BULLSHIT!!!

This is pure BULLSHIT!

You cannot lengthen a muscle. Where a muscle inserts into the tendon and bone is hereditary. The only way you can "lengthen" the muscle would be to surgically have it removed from its insertion point and have it inserted in a different place. Something you certainly don't want to do. What the "experts" are really talking about is making the muscle more flexible. Always do the full range of movement and you will have nothing to worry about. You can also do stretching exercises which will help you to have a greater range of motion.

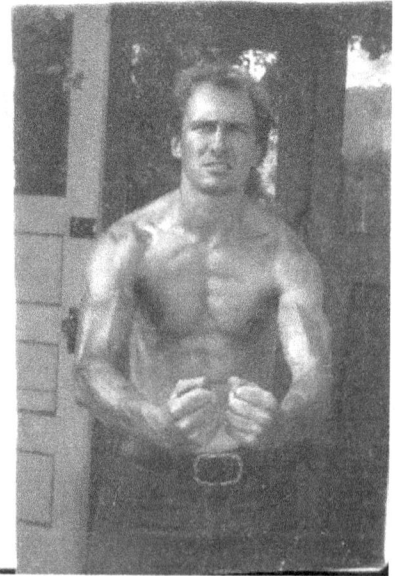

The notion of short bulky muscles is an optical illusion. Take a six foot man who is thin. His muscles will appear to be "long". Add seventy pounds to that man of pure muscle mass and the muscles of his arms will appear to be shorter. Same insertion points of muscle to bone. The muscle, because it is larger, will appear to be shorter.

If you are an ectomorph like I am you will have a challenge gaining a lot of muscle mass and when you do you will have a more "slender" look about you as opposed to a mesomorph who has a larger bone structure and naturally denser muscles. This is hereditary. You can't change your genetic code but you can do wonders working with what you have. My mistake for many years was in thinking I could somehow change my basic genetic code. Work with what you have and develop yourself to the limits of your genetic code. No one can really tell you how far you will go, that is only seen in retrospect. I was told there was no way I would ever be able to gain any muscle size whatsoever by doctors. But just look at the photos. I proved them wrong.

Work out, eat well and let your body find its own level of excellence. You will be amazed at the results!

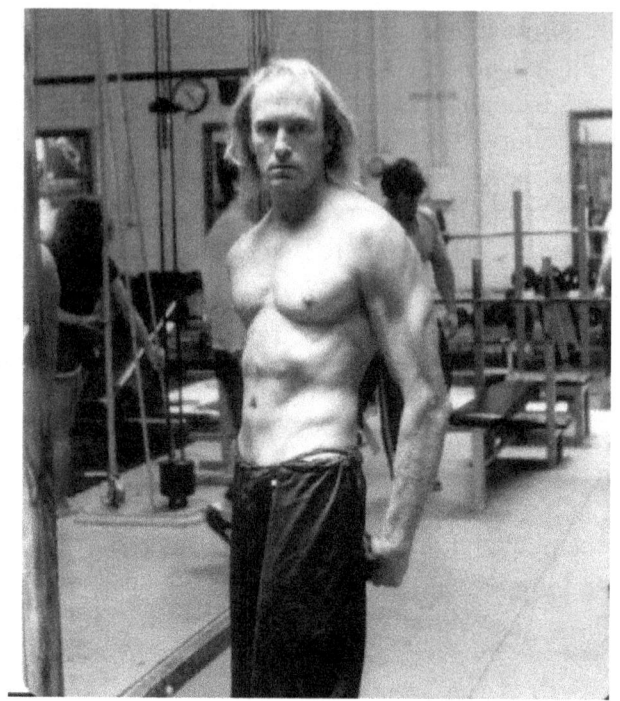

At Gold's Gym, Santa Monica, 1979.
Photo by Al Malone.

CHAPTER TWENTY TWO
"OTHER STRENGTH
TRAINING METHODS"

Are there alternatives to training with weights?

That is a question I am often asked. Can one develop strength and muscle size with other means rather than weights?

First I am going to say this. The best way I know for sure to gain strength and muscle size or even to maintain strength is through training on the basic exercises with barbells and dumbbells. Period!

But there are other ways to build a good physique and I am going to talk about that now.

The Bullworker

The Bullworker is a fantastic exercise device and I own two of them. There are periods when I have worked out with the Bullworker exclusively. And I have had great results. And I have trained a few clients with the device and seen them have great results.

The Bullworker is a spring loaded exercise device that utilizes isometrics, or "static tension". In other words, holding the muscles under tension for a certain length of time, usually ten seconds.

With the Bullworker you can actually do a full body workout in under five minutes!

The advantage of having a Bullworker is space. It's only about two and a half feet long and comes in its own leather carrying case. It can be stored against the wall or under your bed. If you live in a small apartment it won't take up any valuable space. Actually, in my mind, valuable space is space where you would have your weights, bench and squat rack set up in a corner of your room, about an eight by eight square area. But if you don't want to have a bunch of weights in your apartment then the Bullworker is a fantastic way to get in a good strength training workout. Later on in the next chapter I will present a full body workout routine that takes less than five minutes that you can do to get in your strength training requirement. You can order the Bullworker online.

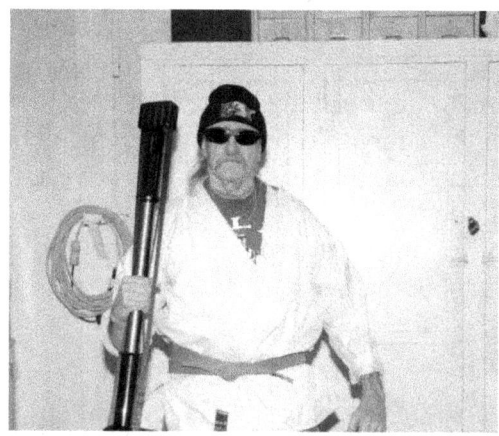

The Bullworker can provide a high intensity workout.
Photo by Randy States.

The Bowflex

Another machine that I have investigated although I have never worked out on is the Bowflex. You can work your entire body on this machine effectively. It can be stored against a wall in your living room and it's quiet. You can do all the basic exercises I have described on it. For apartment dwellers it may be ideal and many use it in combination with treadmills and stationary bikes for a combo of strength training and cardio.

The Total Gym

Another machine I have had experience on is the Total Gym, as advertised by Chuck Norris on his infomercials. He is an avid user of this product. A friend of mine who at the time was hitting seventy had a very muscular physique and I asked him where he worked out at. He told me he worked out at his condo on the Total Gym. He proceeded lead me to his bedroom where he pulled out the machine which was folded up under his bed. It took only a moment to set up and I gave it a try. I got a good pump on several different exercises. It utilizes one's own bodyweight to provide resistance. Resistance can be increased according to the angle you set the machine up on. It provides a very challenging workout. And the great advantage is that it can be easily broken down and stored in a closet or under a bed.

These are the main machines I have actually seen and studied. They provide an effective strength training workout in a minimum of time.

CHAPTER TWENTY THREE
"THE BULLWORKER WORKOUT"

As I said in the previous chapter, I have gotten excellent results using the Bullworker. I have provided photos of myself illustrating a basic routine that actually takes under five minutes. The photos were taken on my 65th birthday back in 2012 by Randy States, a good friend of mine.

I had read about this device way back in 1975 and was mildly curious although, back then, I didn't believe in any strength training methods but weights. I had not yet had my mind opened.

As I have discussed, I learned about the science of recuperation, how the body can take up to seven to fourteen days to recover from a high intensive workout. I have talked about how I discovered that I could get a great workout in and put on muscle mass working out on a heavy basic routine once a week. And the photos of me prove it's true. All this, of course, was done with weights, especially in the basic moves, bench press, squats, deadlifts or powercleans. I have often used machines for the lats, shoulders and arms but usually always I use free weights for bench presses, squats and deadlifts. These are the most effective exercises one can do.

I have often wondered what I would do if I did not have access to weights or a well equipped gym. Some of the gyms I have worked out at include Gold's Gym, Venice. I was a member of Gold's Gym, North Hollywood for a number of years. I also had great workouts at World Gym, Venice although that gym no longer exists. But that is for another story.

I would usually use my motorcycle to get to the gyms but I always, in the back of my mind, wondered what I would do if I could not work out with weights. I had once had a Bullworker given to my by a friend but before I could really try it out to see how effective it was it was stolen. I always had a curiosity about it and regretted losing it. I have done free hand isometrics at times and found them to have a good effect when I couldn't use the weights for a short period of time but these periods were always brief.

So one day I went on line and discovered that the Bullworker was still being sold. About that time I was also given one from a friend at work. I had already sent for a new one so that is how I ended up with two of them.

The Five Minute Experiment

I decided on an experiment to see whether it would be of any real value. A friend of mine named Clint had really been into working out. He had been a skinny guy originally. Then I had noticed that he was putting on muscle. I asked him and he told me that he had started working out with weights. He joined 24 Hour Fitness but then life and responsibilities began to take over and he stopped going. He kept paying his membership but, like millions, he stopped going. He just "didn't have the time". I had always tried to encourage him but he always "had things to do" so he never would go back.

I had the perfect subject. Someone who was "too busy" to train. So I approached him and asked him if he would give the Bullworker a try for six weeks. He said "yes". I also asked him not to go to the gym to work out with weights during the six week period. He said that was "no problem" because he hadn't been to the gym in about two years.

So the experiment was on.

Every Thursday he would come into my office and do a routine that took just under five minutes. I took measurements of his chest and arms and wrote these down.

So every Thursday he would come in to my office and do the following routine. Each isometric hold lasted for twenty seconds.

Chest Crunch
Lat Pull
Shoulder Crush
Curl
Triceps Ext.
Ab Crunch

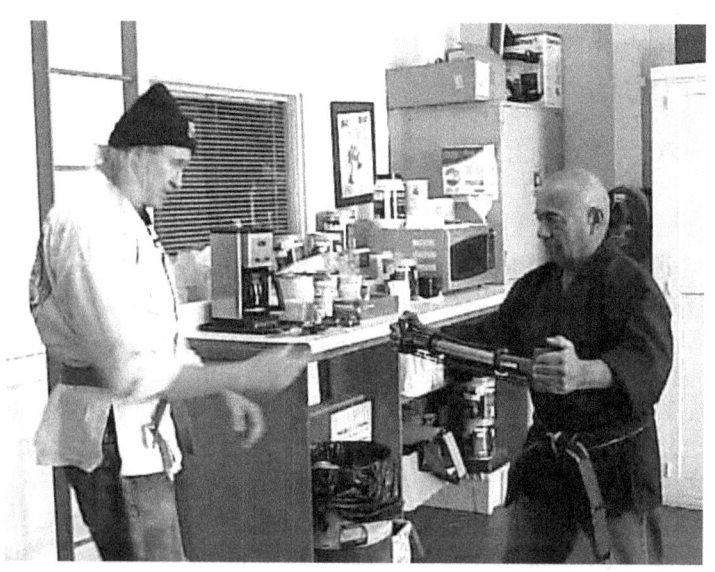

Grand Master Joe Rosas gives the Bullworker a try.

He did this routine for six weeks without failure. At the end of six weeks I took his measurements again and found he had put a half inch on his arms and two inches on his chest!

Wow!

It worked! A five minutes static tension routine once a week and he put on muscle mass. It showed too. He was more defined, cut.

Another friend of mine heard about the experiment. He also wanted to try the Bullworker. He told me that he did endless pushups but that he just couldn't put any size on his chest, no matter what.

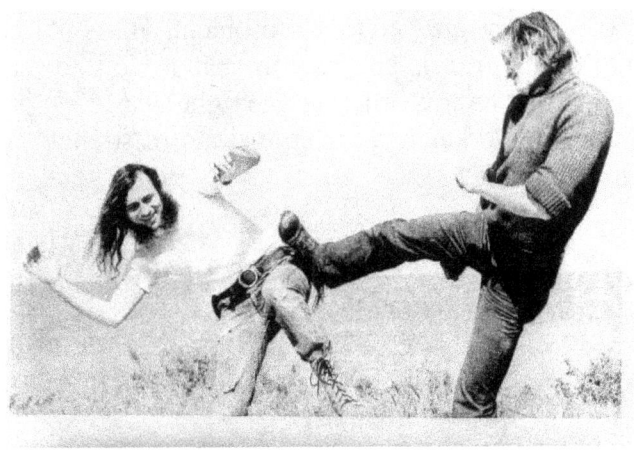

*Starring in the martial arts action movie "*Hammerfist*" in 1975. An Al Malone photo.*

I asked him to give the Bullworker a six week try and also, during that time, to forego the pushups. He agreed and we took his measurements. He did the routine described above for six weeks and got the same results. A half inch on arms and two inches on his chest. Two inches whereas before he had not been able to build any chest size whatsoever! He was delighted with the results.

Seeing it work so well, I kept it in mind and when I was really working a hard schedule, work, school and of course, the writing of my novels, I would do the basic Bullworker workout and it kept my muscle mass in tact. But I would always go back to pumping iron whenever possible.

A vendor came into my office around this time, I could tell he was really into working out. With his short sleeved dress shirt on you could seen that he was very muscular. I asked him if he worked out and he said he did. Swimming twice a week and weights once a week. He expressed regret that because he had to travel so much in his line of work that it was difficult to get a workout in. I showed him the Bullworker and he gave it a try right there in my office. He was so impressed that he said it was the perfect answer to his problem. He could carry it with him on his travels and stay in shape! He told me as he was leaving that he was ordering one right away.

So the Bullworker is a viable method of strength training with limited time.

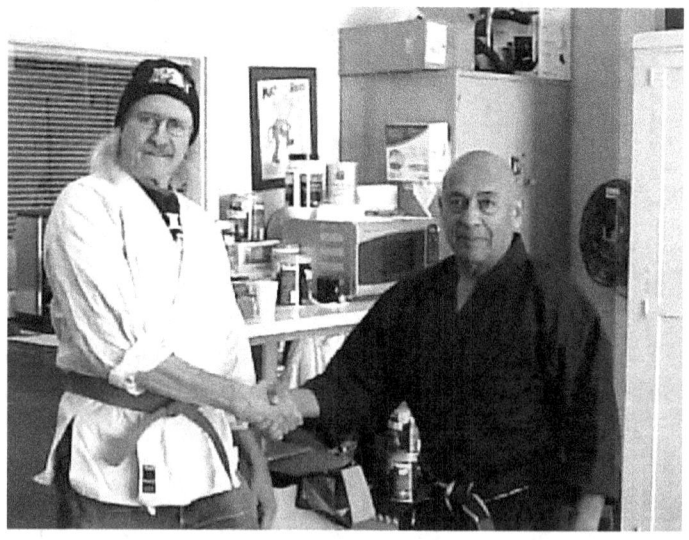

Grand Master Joe Rosas, eighth degree black belt in kenpo karate.

The Exercises

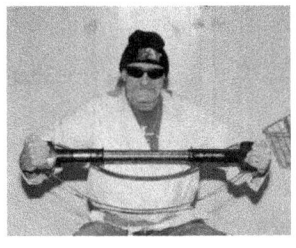

Chest Press

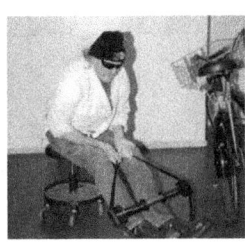

Lat Row

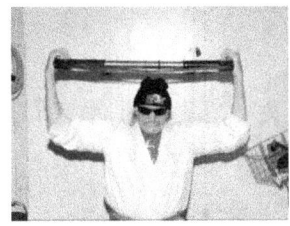

Shoulder Press

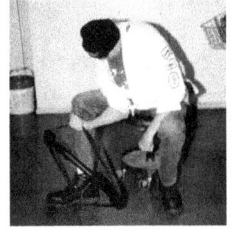

Curl

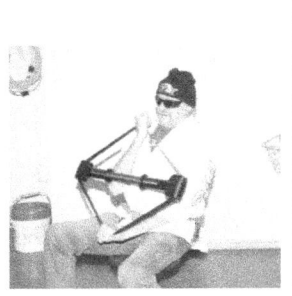

Triceps Extensions

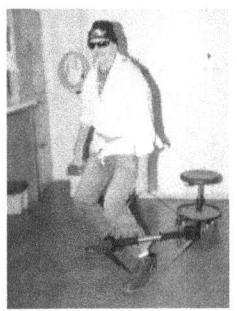

Squats

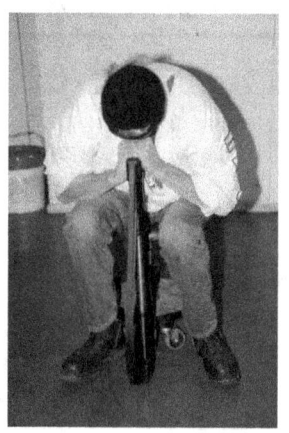

Ab crunch

CHAPTER TWENTY FOUR
"TRAINING PARTNERS"

I usually don't train with a training partner. Many do but I prefer to train alone. But a training partner can be an asset.

I have at times trained with a partner and it was a rewarding experience, usually. But there were other times this was not so. There are certain rules for having a training partner that you should have.

Number one, your training partner should be on the same page. I never train on another person's routine. I have my own ideas on how to train and what works. If someone wants to learn what I know and wants to train with me then I will allow it.

Number two. A training partner must be on time for the workout. I once had a training partner who began showing up late or not at all. I would be waiting for him and getting frustrated. Finally, I told him to be on time or I would start without him. He agreed. The next day, he was not on time so I started the workout. That particular day he didn't even show up! In fact he never showed up again and I didn't even address it with him. I just went right on training. I would see him from time to time and he would talk about getting back into working out but it never happened.

But I have also had valuable experiences with training partners. One partner that comes to mind was Mike O'Brien. He was the youngest of the O'Brien family raised in Marin

County. There were five boys in all, raised by Joe G. O'Brien who was an old time bodybuilding, wrestling and boxing champion, from way back in the old days, the 1930s and forties. He raised his sons on weight training and boxing and they were the toughest kids in Marin County. I got to know the family through my weight training connections.

It was 1974 in my back room gym. I met Mike, the youngest O'Brien one day over at a Kempo Karate school I was working out at and we agreed to start training at my back room gym. So every day at 6:00 pm three days a week, Monday, Wednesday and Friday he would show up and we would work out on the usual basic routine. We pushed each other hard and I could see there were some things he didn't know so I began to teach him. For one thing, he would jerk his curls up. I taught him to slow down and feel the movement. It meant dropping his exercise poundage about twenty pounds. He did and his arms gained an inch and a half in about two weeks! I taught him the proper form in all the exercises and he grew. He was a natural, with the right training program he grew very fast, going from about 180 lbs right up to 210 lbs in about two months. The guy would just look at a weight and grow! He was the strongest of his family.

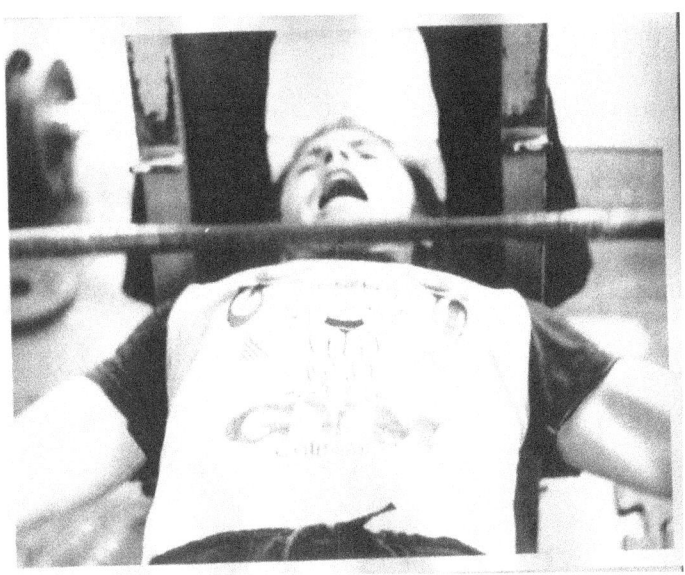

Mike O'Brien does a heavy set on the bench. Scott Gordon Photo.

Another fantastic training partner was Monte Hargraves. He worked at the same place I did, this was in the early nineties and I worked out at a fantastic place called The Power Source. A really hard core gym in Burbank. By this time I was training twice a week and was bigger than I had ever been. We worked out on the basic routine. Bench presses, squats, cable rows, behind the neck presses (an exercise I no longer do or recommend), curls and lying triceps extensions. Two sets each for six to twelve reps.

We changed the routine. On Mondays we would work out heavy, doing many sets of singles on the bench press and squats. On Thursday we would work light, two sets per exercise, doing a "quality workout". Feeling every rep. It was a good program. This lasted more than a year then the gym closed down and we at times trained at other gyms. I joined Gold's Gym, North Hollywood and we would work out there. Monty sustained a hip injury and had to change the way he trained so we no longer trained together as much as his needs were changing.

We still train together occasionally at Gold's Gym, Venice.

I have also had a few other training partners from time to time but they never really hung in so it didn't work out.

So there are advantages and disadvantages to having a training partner.

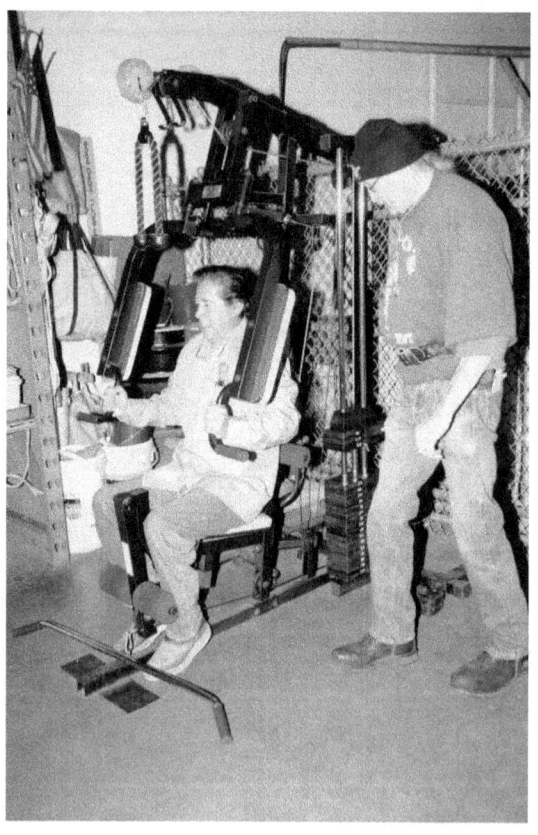

Training partners can shout encouragement.

CHAPTER TWENTY FIVE
"PROPER ORDER"

I want to talk a bit about the proper order of the workout. You want to always work the larger muscle groups first. In other words, don't expend your energy on smaller exercises first as it will take away from your performance in the larger ones.

Don't do exercises like curls and triceps extensions first. You want to put your main energy into the big movements like squats, bench presses, deadlifts and rows. If you work arms first you will not be able to put your full energy into the more important exercises.

If you don't have time to do a full workout you wouldn't want to just do curls. Sitting in front of the TV set doing dumbbells curls is an absolute waste of time. If you want to do one exercise in front of the TV then have a fully loaded barbell in front of your chair. Do the clean and press during commercials. That one single exercise will work almost every muscle in your body.

Doing exercises like dumbbell curls in place of the bigger exercises is just plain laziness! It's a total waste of time, like I just said.

If you have limited time but you can do three exercises then do the squats, bench presses and rows. Between those three exercises the entire body is worked. Squats work legs, but also work the hips and lower back. Bench presses not only work chest, but they also work the shoulders and triceps. And rows not only work the back but also the biceps and forearms. So, those three exercises give your entire body a complete workout.

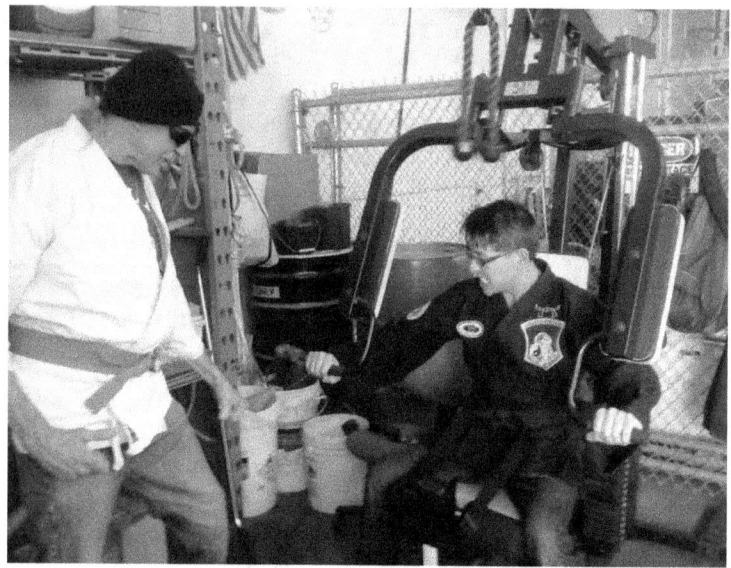

Lambert Cheung, author of the Red Phoenix *trilogy doing machine bench presses.*

Want a short three day a week workout? Monday, do squats. Wednesday do bench presses and Friday do rows. This will work your entire body in a very brief amount of time. When pressed for time I have sometimes just done the Bullworker workout once a week. This is while I was working full time, going to school and also writing novels. That's a pretty busy schedule. So the brief Bullworker workout kept my muscle mass up. Note, I didn't mention cardio. Cardio is valuable but not as valuable as strength training. If I have to choose between the two I always will pick strength training. Cardio does not put the stress on the bones to promote bone density like strength training does. I am sixty eight years old at the time of this writing and have good existing muscle mass along the slender lines that I had in my youth. This would not have happened if I had not dedicated myself to strength training all my adult life. Strength training is vitally important as we age to keep up our quality of life. Because of strength training I have a tremendous quality of life and literally feel like I am eighteen years old!

So never neglect your strength training. It doesn't take a lot time to do.

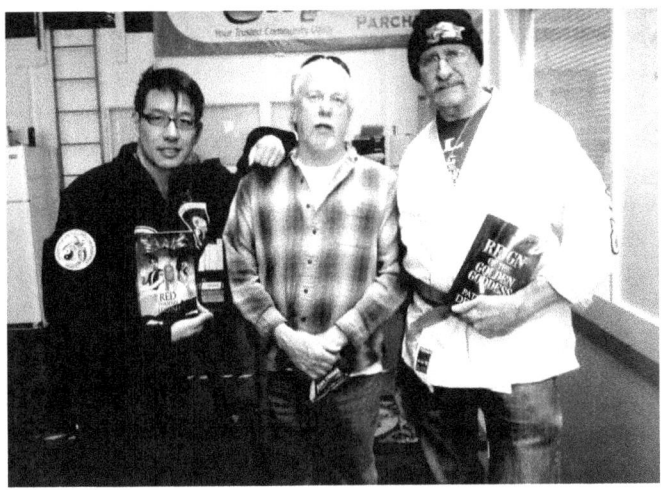

With author Lambert Cheung and training partner Monte Hargraves.

CHAPTER TWENTY SIX
"OTHER ROUTINES"

I am going to present some routines you might want to try. Remember to warm up before the workout.

The Twice a Week Combination

Monday

Bench press 5x5
Squats 5x5
Rows 5x5
Military presses 5x5

Thursday

Dumbell bench presses 2x6-10
Squats 1x20
Stiff legged deadlifts 1x20
Dumbbell rows 2x6-10
Seated dumbbell presses 2x6-10
Seated dumbbell curls 2x6-10
Mallon dips 2x6-10
Always do ab work

The Three Day A Week Split

Monday

Bench presses 2x6-10
Dumbbell or regular rows 2x6-10
Ab work

Wednesday
Squats 1x20
Still legged deadlifts 1x20
Ab work

Friday

Military presses 2x6-10
Curls 2x6-10
Triceps extensions 2x6-10
Ab work

Volume Two Day Split

Ab work to warm up before each session

Monday

Bench presses 5x8
Incline Press 5x8
Lat pulls to chest 5x8
Cable rows 5x8
Seated presses 5x8
Dumbbell presses 5x8
Barbell curls 5x8
Lying triceps extensions 5x8

Thursday

Squats 5x8
Thigh extensions 5x10
Thigh curls 5x10
Seated leg presses 5x10
Stiff legged deadlifts 1x10
Forearm curls each way 1x20-30
Four way neck 1x20 each way

Four Way Split

Monday
Bench presses 2x6-10
Incline presses 2x6-10
Lat pulls to chest 2x6-10
Seated rows 2x6-10

Tuesday

Squats 2x6-10
Thigh extensions 2x6-10
Thigh curls 2x6-10
Stiff legged deadlifts 1x10
Heel raises 2x15

Wednesday, rest

Thursday

Military presses 2x6-10
Dumbbell lateral raises 2x10-15

Friday

Curls 2x6-10

Lying triceps extensions 2x6-10

My Present Routine

Ab crunchs
Leg raises off bench
Good mornings
Bench press 1x6-10
Squats 1x10-20
Dumbbell rows 1x6-10
Standing press 1x6-10
Curls 1x6-10
Lying triceps ext. 1x6-10
Martial arts practice 5 to 10 minutes
Meditation 15 minutes

Questions about the Mallon Dips? An exercise I do that I named after my teacher, Charles P. Mallon. Feet on one bench and palms on another, dumbbell in your lap. Now, dip down and rise back up. Works the triceps.

Good mornings? Not to be done with a heavy weight. This is a warm up exercise. Place a light barbell across the back of your shoulders. Bend at the waist then return to standing position. Do about twenty reps.

The Four Way Neck Exercise: Place the palm of your hand against the side of your head. Now, resisting with your hand, bend your neck to the side. Repeat with the other side. Place both palms on your forehead and while resisting, bend your head forward. Now lock both hands behind your head and while resisting, move your head back. Do fifteen reps each way. This will keep your neck young and supple.

As you can see my routine at the time of this writing is very brief, done with several days rest in between. It keeps me in good shape along with some walking and practicing martial arts exercises.

The routines described here are just a few of the workouts you can do with a limited amount of time. After working out on some of them for a time you will get the idea. You will then become an "instinctive" trainer. As you get to know your body and how it reacts you will begin making up your own routines. Just remember, with limited time, do what's most effective, the big exercises first so you work your main muscle groups. So go to it and good luck! You won't regret it!

CHAPTER TWENTY SEVEN
"I MET A MOVIE STAR"

I met a movie star.

When I was a young teenager back in the 1960s and was training at Charlie Mallon's gym I would watch the Hercules movies on TV on weekends. I had been inspired to lift weights by the movie *Hercules* starring Steve Reeves and they had begun showing the Hercules movies on TV regularly.

One day I was sitting in the office of Charlie's gym looking at the bodybuilding magazines when I saw an article about a bodybuilding champion named Chuck Pendleton. The title of the article was "The Ninth Gladiator". That's because, according to the article, Chuck Pendleton was the ninth American bodybuilder to go to Italy to star in the Hercules, gladiator movies. He was impressive, very muscular and he had a rugged look to him that set him aside from the other bodybuilders who starred in the sword and sandal movies.

I had not seen his movies on TV though. But one Saturday night I saw listed a movie titled *Brennus, Enemy of Rome* starring Gordon Mitchell. I watched the movie and it was Chuck Pendleton, the same man I had seen in the magazines. They had changed his name to Gordon Mitchell for the movies although I don't know what was wrong with the name Chuck Pendleton. A number of Italian bodybuilders had had their screen names changed for the Hercules movies. Actors like Rod Flash, Allen Steel and Kirk Morris. All Italian bodybuilders.

I became a fan of Gordon Mitchell and saw all his movies. The most impressive movie I saw that he made was *Fury of Achilles*. It was quite an inspiring movie.

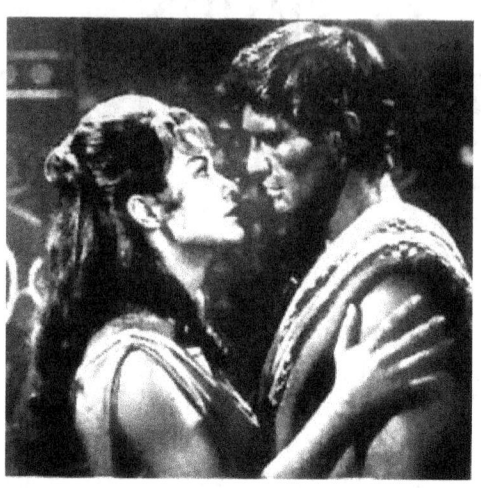

Gordon Mitchell in Fury of Achilles, *1961*
With Gloria Milland, a Medallion Picture, Rome, Italy.

Fast forward to March, 1995.

I was driving west on the 10 Freeway headed for Venice, California. My goal, two choices. I was either going to work out at Gold's Gym or at World Gym which was about three blocks from Gold's. I decided on World Gym and pulled into the parking lot. I went in and paid for a daily workout, $10. The way it worked there was that sometimes they'd let you work out for a day and sometimes they didn't. It depended on the mood of the guy at the desk. I was favored that day but I didn't really know just yet how highly favored I was.

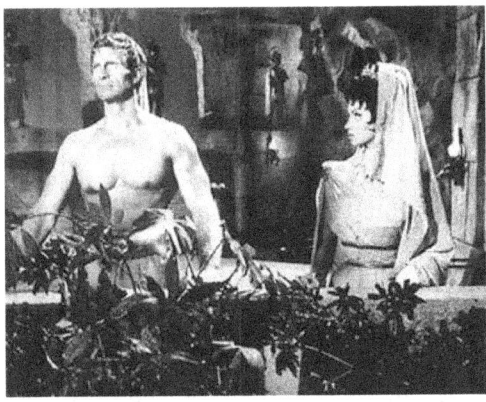

Gordon Mitchell with Chello Alonzo in Atlas in the Land of the Cyclops *, Medallion pictures, Rome, Italy, 1959.*

I suited up and began to train. As I was over at the squat rack I noticed an older man with silver hair and he looked very familiar but I couldn't quite place him. I almost had the name on my lips but still couldn't exactly tell who he was. There was a personnel trainer there named Ira who was training a very muscular female bodybuilder. Ira had been Lou Ferrigno's training partner during the year Lou had been giving his last effort to win the Mr. Olympia title. Ira looked over at the silver haired man and told the woman he was training, "Chuck, over there, he's a movie star."

Immediately a light went on in my brain!

Standing there on the training room floor was the man himself, Chuck Pendleton, Gordon Mitchell! I was simply amazed. There was the man whose movies I had seen as a kid. I remember taking the bus all the way over to San Francisco just to see his movies. And now, here he was, right there on the gym room floor.

"Wow!" I said to myself. "I gotta meet this guy!"

He was just about to start walking up the steps to the locker room. This was my last chance!

"Sir," I said.

"Yes," he answered as he paused.

"You're Chuck Pendleton aren't you?"

"Yes," he said.

"My name is Pat and I used to watch your movies!"
I came forward and he smiled and we shook hands.

"And you have another name?" he said.

"Pat Deu Pree," I blurted out.

"And what do you do?"

I told him I worked for a large southern California utility. Then he said, "I am here on Fridays and Saturdays from noon to three. When you come here at that time you shall be my guest here."

I was utterly dumbfounded! Wow! To actually train at World Gym as the guest of Gordon Mitchell! What a gift! I was greatly favored that day.

For the next eight years I would visit Gordon and take a workout at World Gym from time to time. During that time I realized my mission in life was to be a fiction writer and I even co-wrote a book with Gordon, *MUSCLE BEACH*, a fictionalized science fiction novel about a communist plot to set off an atomic bomb in Santa Monica bay set in the 1950s with Gordon Mitchell as a bodybuilding private detective. He gave me all the background of that era in the history of Muscle Beach for he had lived it. The novel never did see publication although we gave it a good run. I also wrote a screenplay for the novel. I had never written a screenplay before and Gordon taught me the ropes. He was a great inspiration to me. He passed from this earth in September, 2003. He had just turned eighty years old.

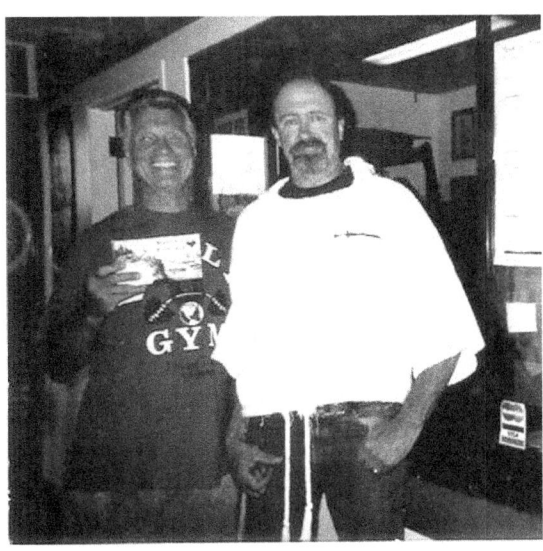

With Gordon Mitchell at World Gym, Venice, 1995.

Through my journey in strength training I have met many life long friends. It's been a fulfilling life. There were jobs I never would have been able to do without the strength that I was able to develop from weight training. Without the endurance I was able to build. I have had many opportunities in life that would not have been possible if I had not picked up a weight way back when I was that skinny, weak seventeen year old kid.

Through weight training I was able to develop a strong will. Without that strong will power I would never have been able to write and publish eleven novels, or go to school, all while working full time.

I have never been too busy to take the time to train. I have never used the excuse that "I was just too busy". Actually, I become really angry whenever I hear that excuse.

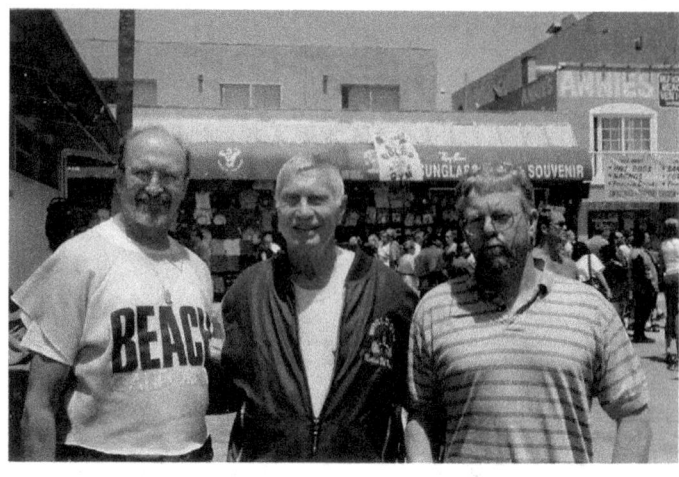

With Gordon Mitchell and my training partner, Monte Hagraves at the Memorial Day Muscle Beach Classic in 2001 where Gordon received a lifetime achievement award.

I have presented here in these pages a formula you can use to fit a workout into any schedule. Whether it's three times a week, or as I have proved, once a week, you can benefit from strength training. I always have preferred weight training with barbells and dumbbells but I have also told you about other methods of strength training that work. It's really up to you, which method to choose. I have also told you about the benefits of meditation. I highly recommend the Transcendental Meditation program but I have shown you the other methods of mediating should you choose to use those.

So, from intense action through weight training to deep rest and relaxation from meditating I have shown you ways to greatly improve your life.

There it is. It's up to you. I have greatly enjoyed sharing this journey with you and I hope you will give strength training a try. You won't regret it.

And always remember, honor your teachers.

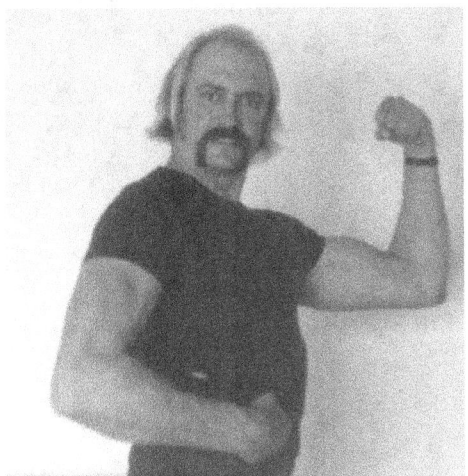

Photo by Amanda Torres.

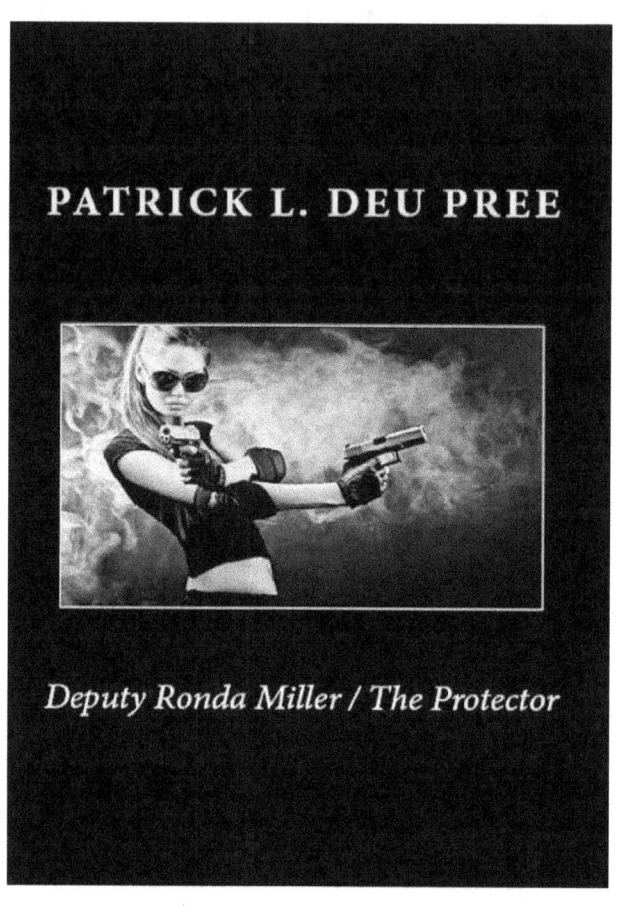

PATRICK L. DEU PREE

Deputy Ronda Miller / The Protector

Don't get in her way!
Intense, high octane adventure from
Patrick L. Deu Pree

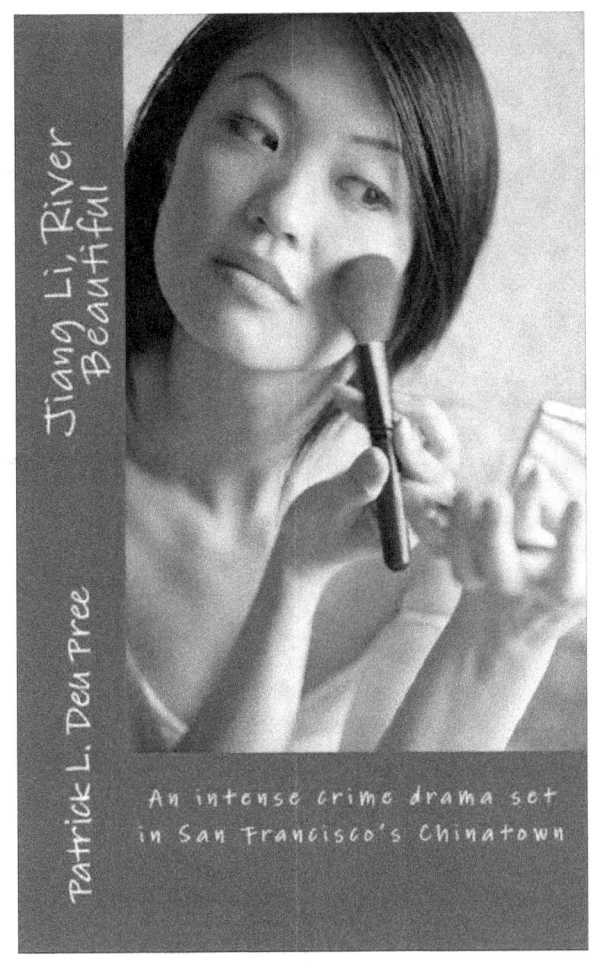

Jiang Li, River Beautiful

Patrick L. Den Pree

An intense crime drama set in San Francisco's Chinatown

Crime and romance in San Francisco's Chinatown!

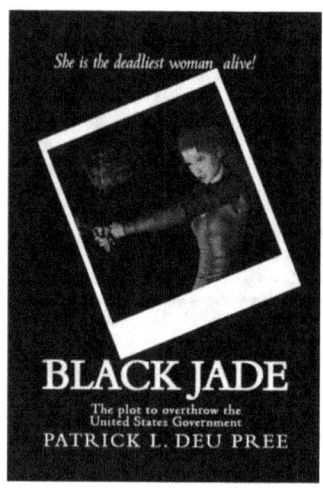

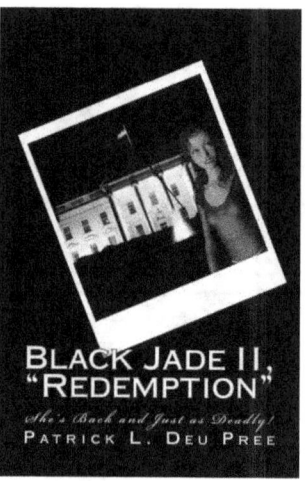

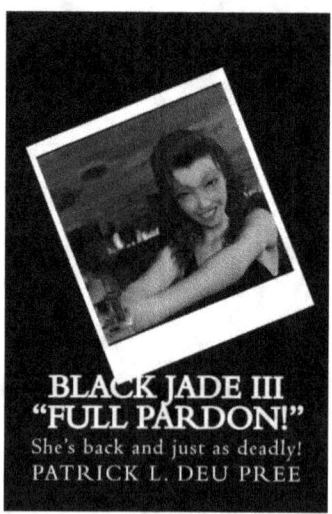

The Black Jade Trilogy!

The Kshatriya series by
Patrick L. Deu Pree

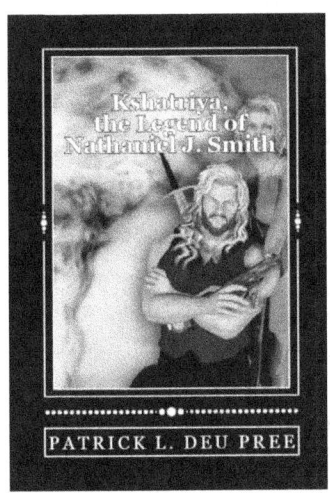
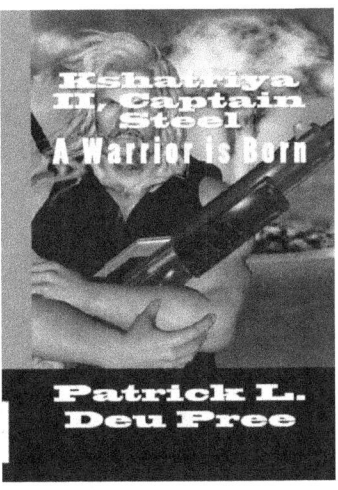

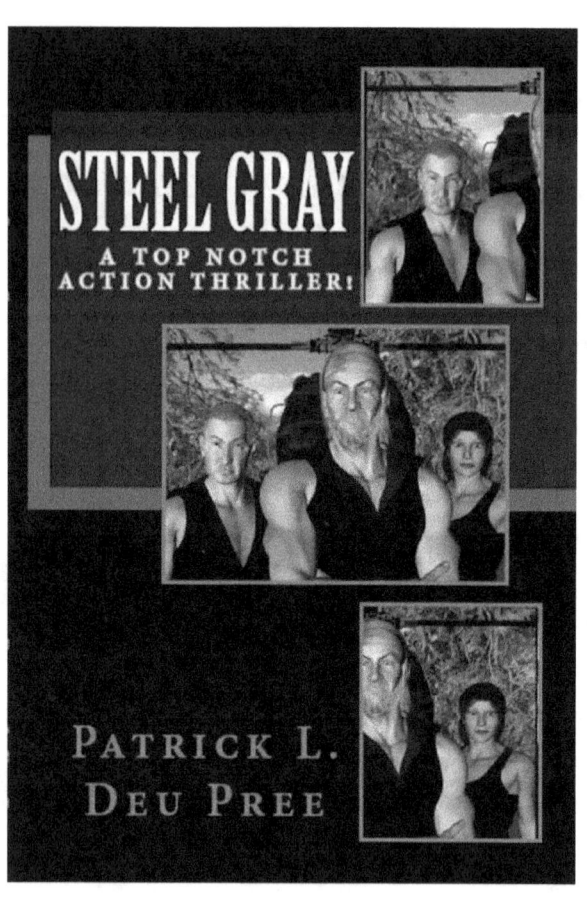

Revenge and Justice in modern day Vietnam!

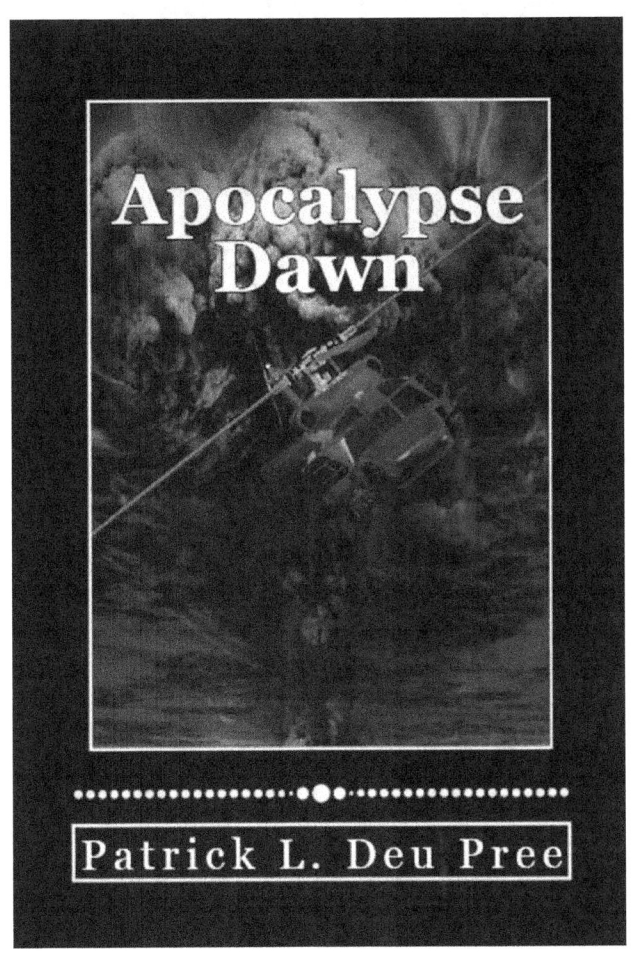

A Vietnam era thrillride!!

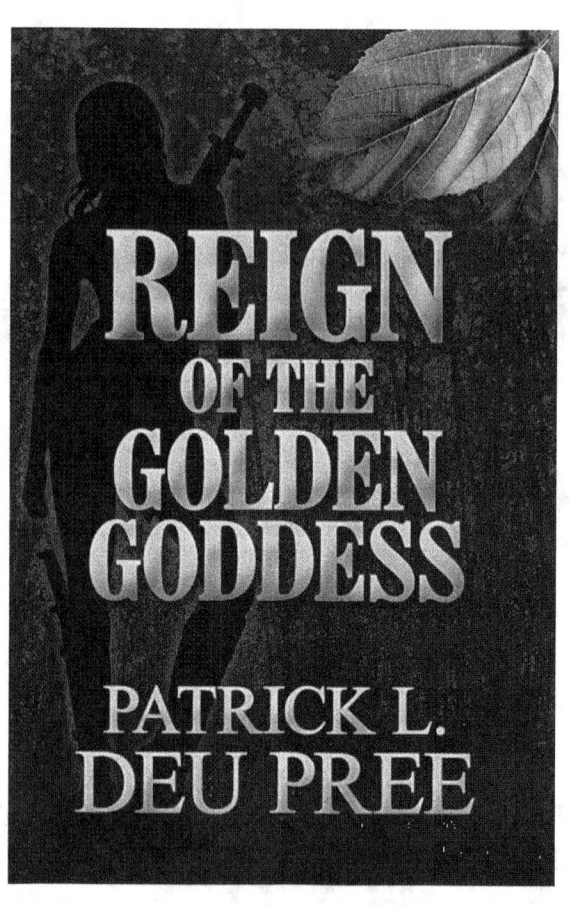

Natalie Jayne Smith, daughter to Kshatriya's Nathaniel J. Smith, faces her greatest challenge as she is transported to a mythical kingdom 10,000 in the past!

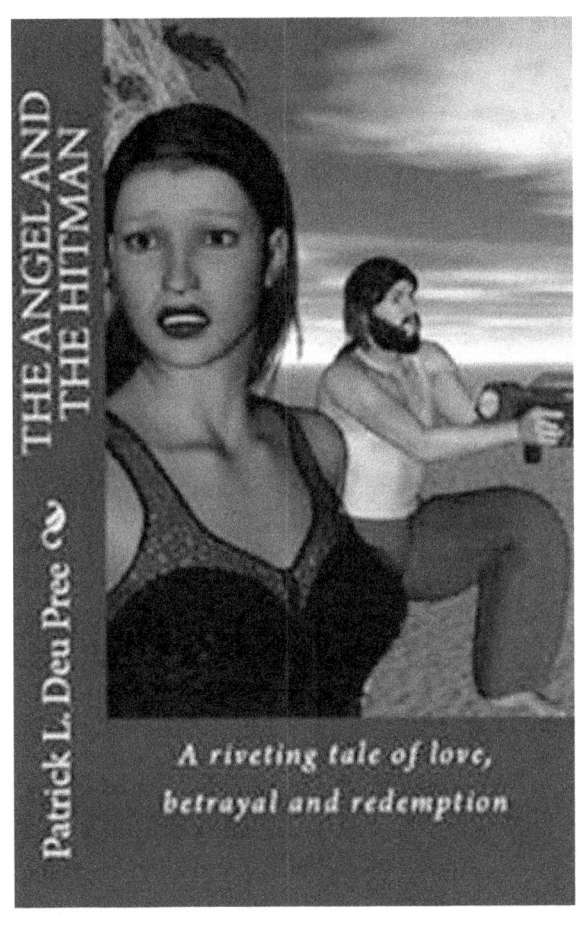

A woman with unusual powers and the man sworn to protect her!

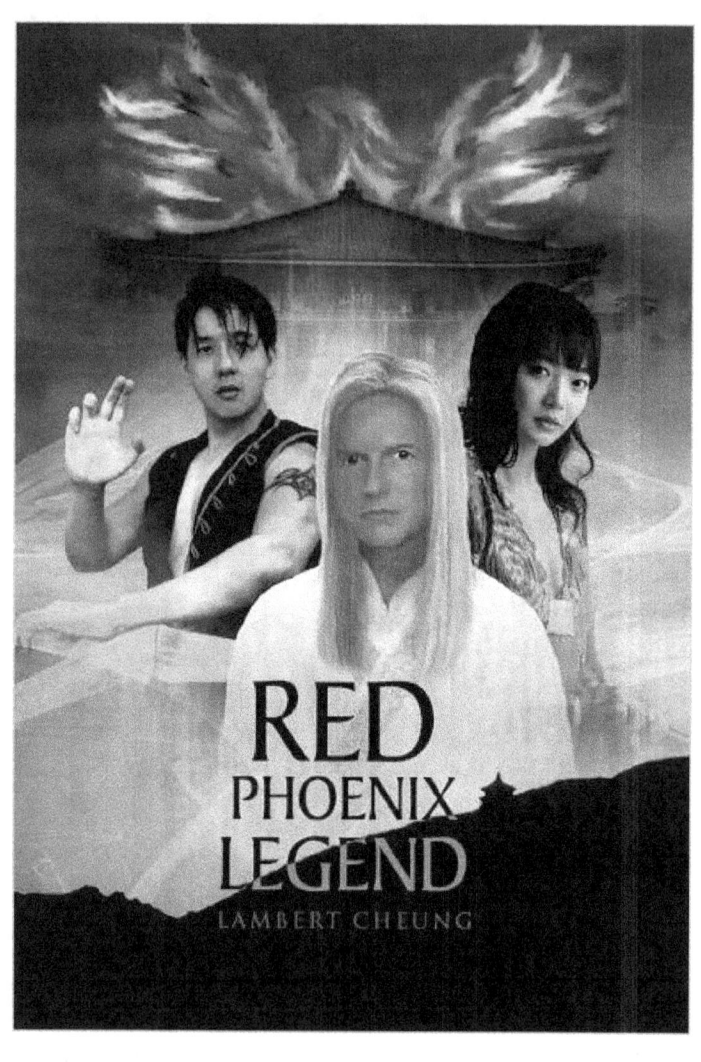

RED
PHOENIX
LEGEND

LAMBERT CHEUNG

Don't miss this fantastic action filled thriller by Lambert Cheung!

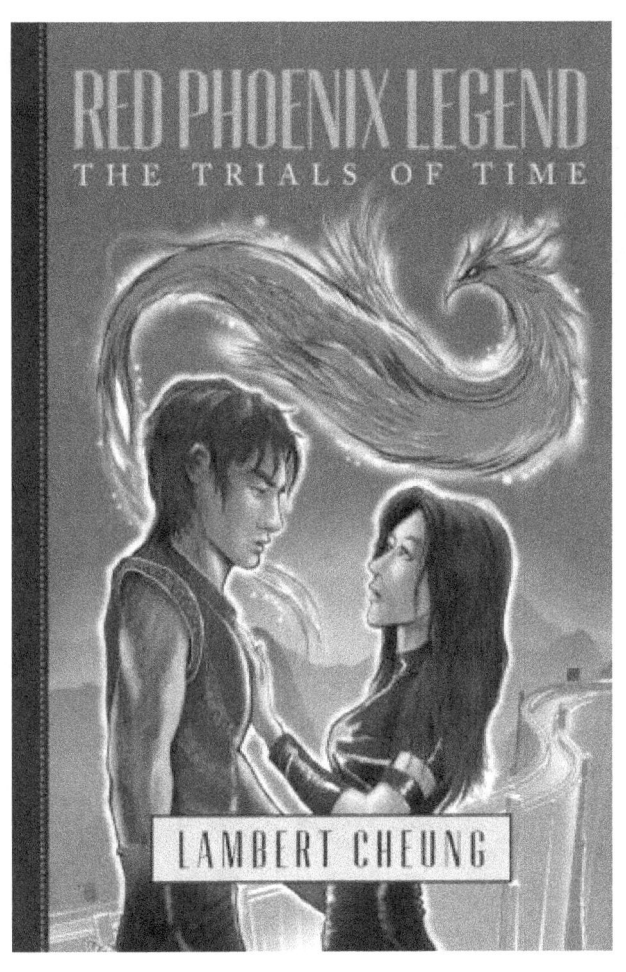

Another fantastic thrill ride from Lambert Cheung!

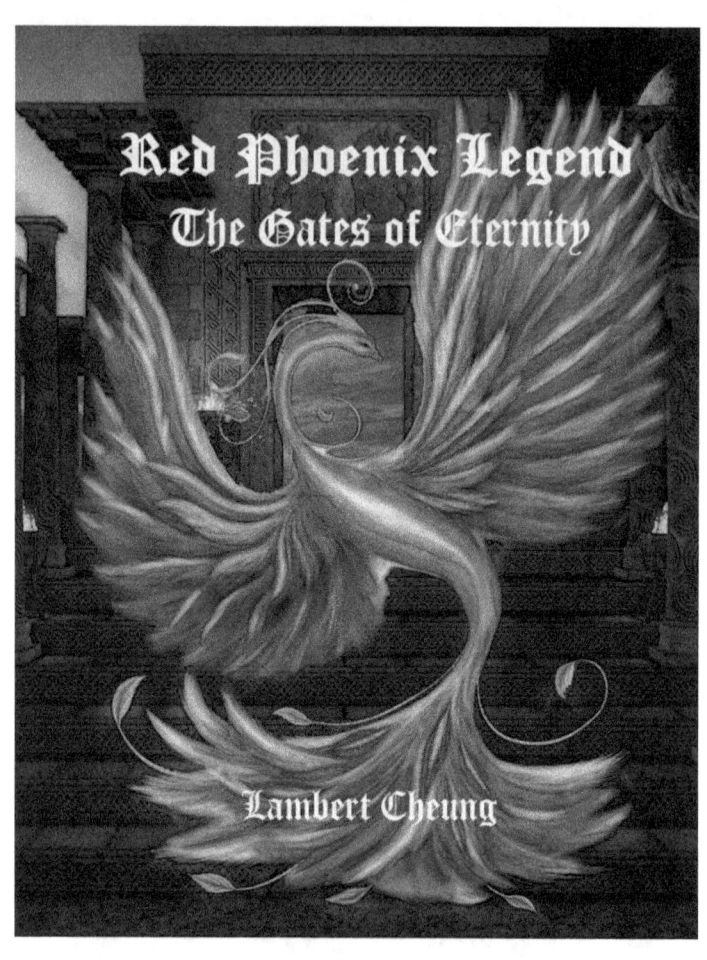

Coming soon from Lambert Cheung! Don't miss this third in the Red Phoenix trilogy!